STRATEGIES FOR ALCOHOL AND OTHER DRUGS TREATMENT IN LOW RESOURCE SETTING IN INDIA

Authors

Dr Gargi Sinha

Dr Nilotpal Das

Dr Gargi Sinha

MBBS (Lady Hardinge Medical College, Delhi)

Grad Dip Public Health (Edith Cowan University, Australia)

Dr Nilotpal Das

MBBS ,MD (AIIMS, Delhi, India)

Fellow of Australian and New Zealand College of Psychiatrists (FRANZCP Australia)

TABLE OF CONTENTS

TABLE OF FIGURE

1.0 Objectives

- Describe the clinical presentation of various drug uses in the community

- Outline strategies for harm minimisation of drug

- Distinguish between acute and chronic symptoms of substance use

- Understanding various terminologies used in substance use

- Outlining treatment options available for individual and support for family

- The recovery process for addiction

2.0 Introduction

The excessive use of alcohol and other drugs is becoming an urgent public health challenge for India's rural community. Recent data of a national survey showed a significantly high prevalence of alcohol consumption and skyrocketing prevalence of illicit drugs. Although traditionally, India's rural population would use rice made liquor and cannabis. However, with the availability of illicit drugs such as amphetamine tablets and opioids such as heroin and codeine cough syrup are showing an upward trend among the young generation. The proliferating trend of alcohol and drug use among young people is linked deeply to the biological factors such as dependence on the substance and social factors such as social disintegration and youth unemployment. Hence, to reduce the burden of substance use, healthcare providers need to understand the model of addiction from the biopsychosocial angle and collaboratively work with the individual and the community.

While there is a wide range of evidence to suggest medical treatment of substance use disorder; however, there is a significant dearth of resources about the integrated model of care for substance use disorder designed to meet the low resource setting demands. Hence, the manual has tried to give an overview of the grass root strategies for management of addiction in a low resource setting.

3.0 Problem Statement

While addressing alcohol and drug use in India's underdevelopment region, it is essential to understand the magnitude of the problem nationwide in India. According to a recent national survey conducted by the Government of India, alcohol is the most widely used substance throughout the nation. The estimation by the national report suggests that around 16 crore people in India consume alcohol. Despite being a small state, Tripura remains one of the excessive alcohols using states; more than 10% alcohol of alcohol users are dependent drinker. In terms of treatment, the national recommendation states that 1:3 of alcohol users in India require treatment; however, only 1:40 receives support and treatment for addiction. Hence, the focus should on the training of healthcare providers working in the remote regions of India.

In terms of other drugs, cannabis remains the second most common substance used in India, approximately three crores of the Indian population using cannabis at any given point of time. Its use has been higher in the North-eastern states, UP and Punjab. 1 in 10 is dependent users, and 1:3 requires help. Another widely used substance in India is opioid. Opioids are the third most common addictive substance used in India. Most used opioid is heroin, followed by pharmaceutical opioids, such as codeine cough syrups, opioid pain medication. While just over two crores Indian population uses opioids, the North-eastern states, UP and Punjab, are the highest users. Hence, to reduce the burden of alcohol and other drugs use the emphasis should be on the availability of training and treatment programs and the community's participation for the uptake of preventing strategies.

4.0 Factors influencing substance use

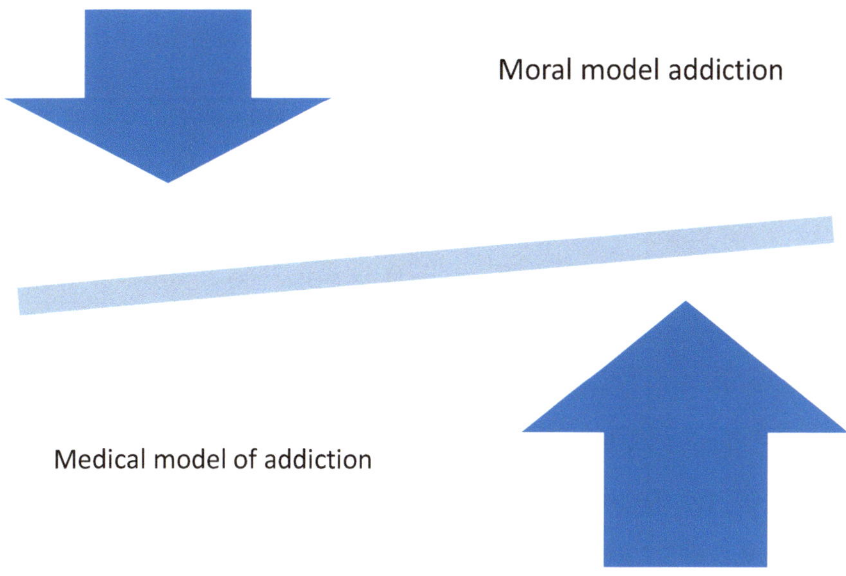

Figure 4.1

There is a large body of evidence that suggests that Alcohol and drug use usually create negative attitudes in our society. Nowadays, it is a common scenario while we pick up a newspaper or turn on the television set and hear a story about how dangerously an addict acted under the influence of some addictive substance. Our beliefs and attitudes have been significantly influenced by the news displayed by our media and society's beliefs. Our society views drug addiction with two opposing ideologies: the 'moral' model of addiction and the 'disease' model of addiction. The moral model of addiction entails addiction is a personal choice and is a moral or will power failure. In contrast, the disease model of addiction describes an addiction as a disease with a multifactorial origin.

When addiction is perceived as a moral problem or will power weakness, individuals with addiction problems tend to face punitive consequences and social stigmatization instead of treating their condition. On the other hand, if addiction is considered as a medical illness, there is much less stigma. As a result, addiction problem is discussed as an issue of medicine rather than the criminal justice system. Drug addiction is identical to other

 chronic illnesses in terms of its onset and trajectory of the illness that is influenced by psychological, social, and environmental factors and genetic determinants.

The proponents of the moral model of addiction blame individuals. The blaming attitude of society helps them to shrug off their responsibility as a member of society. Unfortunately, it produces a culture of denial and ignorance. This attitude produces significant stigma in society about substance use. It is possible to change the culture of victim-blaming and genuinely give an addict a chance to seek treatment for their problem. Research has shown that victim-blaming is one of the major obstacles for overcoming addiction problems. The blaming attitude of the community often dissuades addicts from seeking help due to embarrassment. This attitude can be overcome by involving the community in the treatment of an addict.

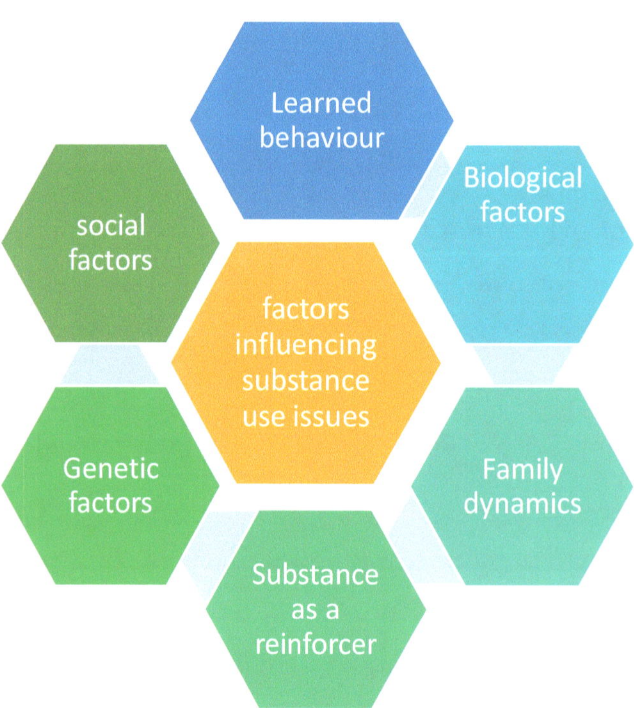

Figure 4.2

Substance dependence results from a complex interaction among multiple biopsychosocial factors. Presence of risk factors is not enough to develop dependence, but the interaction between various risk factors is critical for its development.

- **Biological factor-** Genetic factor plays a crucial role in the intergenerational transmission of an addictive disorder, particularly alcohol. One large family study showed that around 50% of siblings of an alcoholic person met the criteria the diagnosis of alcohol dependence in their lifetime. Certain communities have more tolerance to alcohol due to faster metabolism of alcohol by aldehyde dehydrogenase due to some genetic variation.

- **Family dynamic-** Conflictual family environment provides a fertile ground for addiction. The focus of parental conflict is displaced on the addicted child, which unconsciously maintains the family's homeostasis. Research showed a high incidence of parental domestic violence and divorce in alcohol use disorder population. Overprotective mother and emotionally distant father also predispose children to addiction. Parental neglect and childhood abuse are a risk factor addiction a well.

- **Social factor-** Certain social factors play an important role in initiating and sustaining substance addiction. For instance, parental role modelling, which means young people learn from their parents. If they see their parents using substances, they are more likely to experiment with it. Another issue is peer group approval. People of the adolescent age group usually strive for approval from their friends. They try to shape their individual's identity through appreciation of their peer group. They are usually introduced to substance for the first time in the teenage as a social lubricant. Additionally, social acceptability theory explains that substance use habit usually starts with socially sanctioned substances. Some substances, such as alcohol, is socially acceptable in many cultures. Gradually, alcohol introduces them to other hard drugs. Furthermore, the cost of substance, availability of substance, availability, and acceptability of addiction treatment services in the community also determine addiction.

- **Reinforcer-** All positive reinforcements mediated via the dopaminergic system. Dopaminergic neural pathways are originating from the ventral tegmental area and nucleus accumbens in the brainstem. For chronic users, the glutamatergic system of the brain is more predominantly involved. NMDA receptors in the brain are upregulated due to chronic use of the substance. Thus, substance withdrawal state in the dependent users is due to hyperexcitability of upregulated NMDA receptors.

- **Psychological factor**- Social learning theory describes peer group approval as a motivating factor for addiction. In other words, young people often begin to use the substance to socialise with their friends. Unfortunately, with ongoing use of the substance, their recreational nature turns into a habit called substance dependence. Operant conditioning theory explains how young people use the substance as a self-medication strategy to cope with their underlying psychological issues. Research suggests that mental illness and substance use disorder can co-exist in 50% of cases. Additionally, classical conditioning illustrates how drug paraphernalia merely sees some substance use devices may trigger the strong craving for using the substance.

5.0 Dimension of addiction

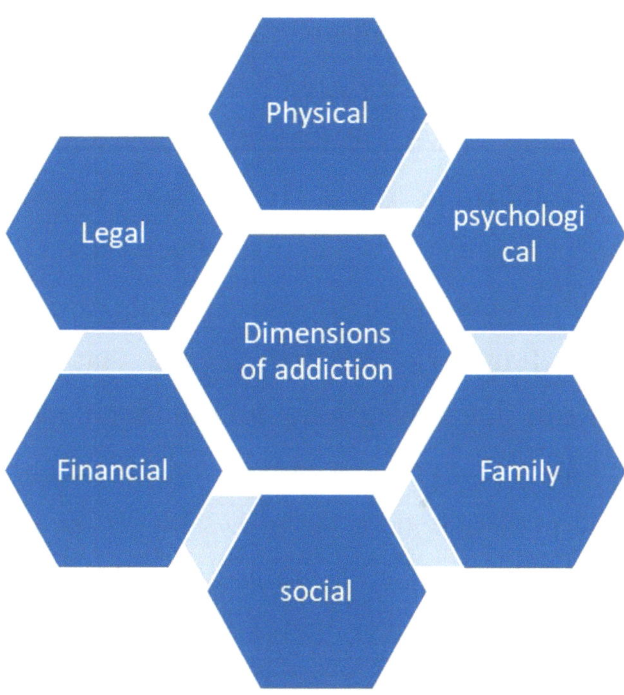

Figure 5.1

5.1 Family of addict

The addiction recovery process is a challenging proposition for the spouses, who often feel powerless when the partner uses substances inspite of all their efforts. Their emotional roller coaster continues considering the persistent risk of relapse. Addictive disorder poses significant stress and trauma to the family members, particularly the spouse. The spouse may switch between being a rescuer who tries to fix all the problems and a demoralised family member who feels helpless and wants peace. Spouses often have frustration built up after years of going through the cycle with their addicted spouse. An addict's spouse feels a great deal of shame and helplessness to break the cycle of addiction.

Creating a boundary between supportive and enabling behaviour is essential. Generally, by keeping silent about the addicted partner's substance use behaviour, a spouse can send the wrong message that they approve the partner's drug dependency. It can be overwhelming to think about drawing boundaries and discussing how their drug use is hurting them. However, at times, this is the only way to break the cycle of co-dependency.

Similarly, it is devastating for parents to watch their adult children getting traps in the cobweb of addiction. As parents of an addicted person, they have cared for and raised their children to their best ability, and it is challenging for them to see their children going down the spiral because of addiction. In most of the cases, parents of substance-using children dedicate their life to raise them. When their children deviate into the pathway of addiction, they feel incredible shame and stigma around it. Parents of addicts often fall into the trap of overprotecting their children, hoping that they will change their behaviour. As a result, parents unknowingly end up enabling their children's behaviour, and their children cannot learn from their mistakes, and their behaviour indirectly gets reinforced. Therefore, the addiction monster grows bigger in their children. Family members silently bear the brunt of addiction, while our society and government seldom think about their plight in the journey of addiction. However, family members also need necessary support from the community and government to rebuild their lives.

5.2 Children of addict

Lisa Frederiksen, a daughter of an alcoholic mother, coined the term 'Second-hand Drinking' (SHD) to refer to the negative impact of alcoholic parents on their children. Approximately 1 in 3 children of parents with addiction develops an addiction problem in their adult life. They are introduced to the substance at a much earlier age than other children with normal childhood upbringing. Sadly, innocent children of addicts become an unprecedented victim of immense psychological trauma. Living with addict parents resembles living in the war zone, where family dynamic revolves around chaos and unpredictable behaviour of addicts. To avoid confrontation with substance users, children often pretend that everything is normal in their home. This causes a severe psychological impact, especially on the family's vulnerable members, such as children. They experience significant shame and guilt but remain either in denial or being a silent spectator. However, they are generally not allowed to share their family secret with others. Thus, children learn to live with psychological pain.

Parental attitude towards their child usually forms the foundation of a parent-child dyadic model called 'attachment'. Childhood attachment usually influences their personality development in later life. Childhood attachment also influences their thinking process and behaviour of other people in their life. Children's early experiences with the parents make the foundation of their future behaviour and determine how they will relate to others. In the absence of stable attachment, children develop a fragile self-image, making them vulnerable to significant mental health problems in the future, such as depression, addiction, and personality disorder. Children may develop post-traumatic stress disorder after witnessing domestic violence between their intoxicated parents. They often miss out in studies and get deviated from career trajectory. Their life gets halted in a stage when normal children endeavour to develop their self-esteem, personality, social skills, and sense of trust within themselves. Despite receiving addiction treatment, they find it hard to have a regular life in society. They remain socially isolated and pose a significant risk of relapse to substance use in future.

Another phenomenon observed in children of an addict is that they play the role of their parent. Adults who suffer from addiction are unable to attend their duties and responsibilities. Once a child takes responsibility for their addict parents, they suffer from terrible consequences. They often do it at the cost of their own developmental needs. Such phenomena are called 'Parentification', which was coined by Boszormenyi-Nagy and Spark. Parentification compromises needs of children. For example, kids of parents who have a serious addiction problem are forced to grow up too early and often learn to ignore and neglect their own needs. The parentification poses an enormous risk to children which go beyond their school life. It threatens psychological health and development throughout life, including identity development, personality, interpersonal relationships, and relationships with an individual's children affected.

Even though the impact of addiction on children is significantly damaging, there are only limited services available in India that address parental addiction's impact on the family's vulnerable children. Sadly, our education system is not sensitive enough to detect and nurture this group of traumatised little souls. It will need the hour to detect this high-risk group of children and help them stay on the track to prevent a downward spiral in their later life.

5.3 Legal issue

Drug addicts may come in the attention of the criminal justice system for several reasons: A person who is possessing illicit drugs might have committed in drug dealing offence. Drug addicts may be involved in legal services due to violent episode under the influence of a substance. It is not uncommon for drug addicts to be charged for various antisocial behaviours to sustain their drug habits. They are often involved in road traffic violation issues leading to legal charges.

6.0 Signs of addiction

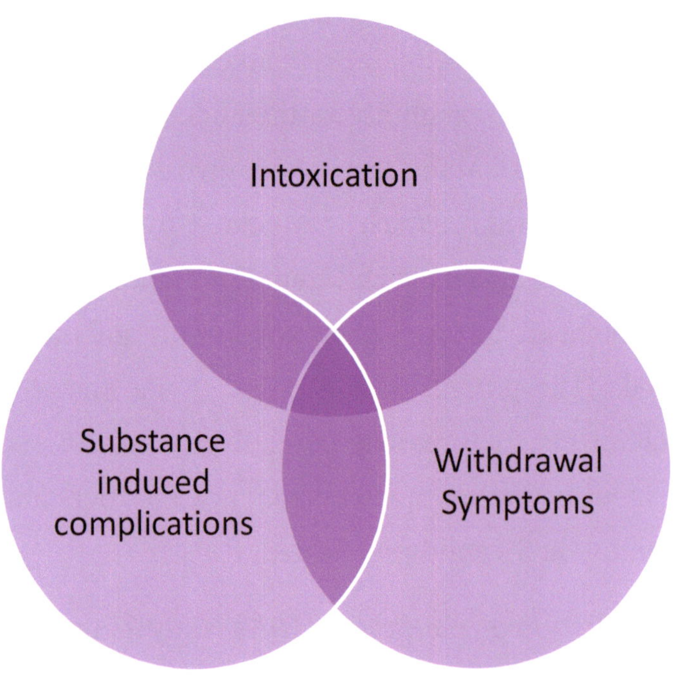

Figure 6.1

Thorley's Model of substance addiction

A British psychiatrist, Anthony Thorley (1982) proposed three patterns of alcohol use associated with alcohol-related harm. For instance, intoxication, regular use, and dependent use. Acute intoxication can cause physical injuries to the person and to others. Regular use means using substance above the safe limits on most of the days. Even a small amount of substance use over an extended period can increase risk of cancer and other short- and long-term health complications. For instance, chronic alcohol use is a well-established risk factor for cancer. Dependent users mean people are investing more and more time to procure substance to avoid discomfort experienced without the substance. The percentage of the dependent users are very low. Thorley's model emphasizes that substance related harm not only arises from dependent level of use but also from single episode of intoxication and small amount of use on a regular basis.

Substance use patterns can be classified as following:

Experimental use- It is usually motivated by the desire to experience a new feeling/mood in company of a group of friends who are also experimenting with the substance.

Social/recreational use- It usually means using substance in a well-controlled way in a social setting/situation.

Circumstantial use- It means using substance to serve some specific purpose, such shift worker, long-route truck driver and performance enhancement in the sports.

Binge use- It means using a large amount of substance at a time to get extra high or to escape from some life stressor.

Regular use- It means using substance in moderation but usually above the safe limit over an extended period. Regular use usually serves some purpose, such as enhancement of sleep, lifting of mood, etc.

Compulsive use- This is also called dependent use. People feel compelled to use substance to avoid distress caused by withdrawal symptoms. They also use drugs at the cost of range of other important activities. This group people are unable to stop using substance despite experiencing significant physical, social, and mental health consequences.

6.1 Cannabis

Marijuana or cannabis refers to the dried leaves, flowers, stems, and seeds from the Cannabis plant. The plant consists of tetrahydrocannabinol and other similar compounds. People smoke marijuana in hand-rolled cigarettes or in pipes or water pipes. Some cannabis preparation can be consumed orally as well.

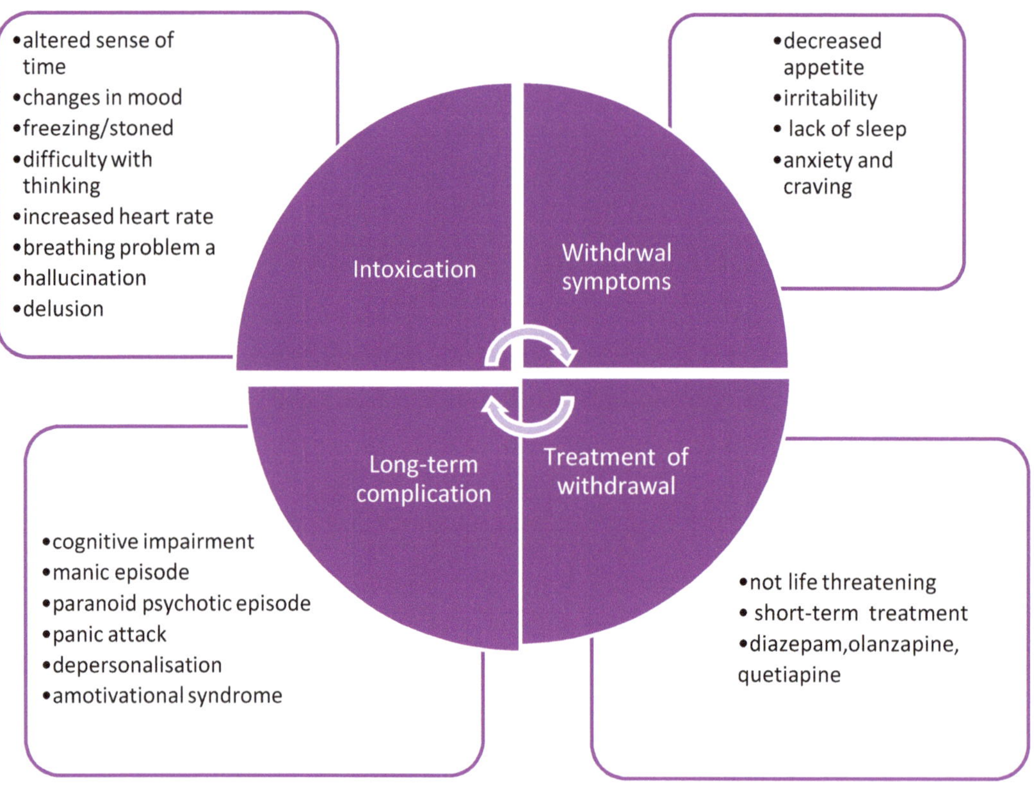

Figure 6.1.1

Long term effects of cannabis

i.   Cognitive impairment- A study from New Zealand (Meier MH et al 2012) showed that people who started smoking cannabis heavily in their teens lost an average of 8 IQ points between ages 13 and 38. Their lost mental abilities did not fully return in those who quit marijuana as adults. Those who started smoking marijuana as adults did not show notable IQ declines.

ii. Manic/Psychotic episode- Acute psychosis can be precipitated by high potency cannabis but cannabis has no causal association with chronic schizophrenia like psychosis. It can exacerbate symptoms of existing psychotic condition, such as schizophrenia. People become quite suspicious and hear voices or see things when no one is around them. They may also feel a bit manic under cannabis intoxication which is characterised by a super happy state of mind, feeling like over the top, talking fast and doing things completely out of their character.

iii. Anxiety related symptoms- Anxiety attack, and depersonalisation/derealisation experience. People experiences a dream like state, as if things around them are not real.

iv. Amotivational syndrome – It is associated with chronic cannabis use, characterised by apathy, poor concentration, social withdrawal, and loss of interest in their pursuits.

v.   Children exposed to marijuana in the womb have an increased risk of problems with attention, memory, and problem-solving compared to unexposed children. Some research also suggests cannabis excreted into the breast milk of nursing mothers could affect the baby's developing brain.

Cannabis withdrawal symptoms

- Many people who use cannabis for many years' experience withdrawal symptoms, when they try to come off the drug.

- It is characterised by decreased appetite, irritability, lack of sleep, anxiety, and craving.

- Symptoms may last one to two weeks.

- There are no significant complications of withdrawal that would necessitate inpatient treatment.

There are no specific medications for cannabis withdrawal symptoms, but medications can be used for short-term symptomatic treatment. For instance, diazepam 5-40mg for 7-10 days, olanzapine 2.5 mg to 10mg for 7-10 days and quetiapine 25mg to 100mg for 7-10 days.

Psychotic symptoms should be managed with an antipsychotic medication such as olanzapine or risperidone for up to 2-3 months or more depending on the severity of symptoms.

6.2 Opioid addiction

Opioid addiction is commonly seen in persons who are being prescribed on opioid pain medications, such as oxycodone, dextropropoxyphene. Heroin is an opioid drug made from morphine; a natural substance taken from the various opium poppy plants' seed pod. Heroin can be white or brown powder. Another name of heroin is smack. People can inject, sniff, snort, or smoke opioids. Some people mix heroin with crack cocaine; a preparation called a speedball. Opioids are highly addictive drugs. Those people who use opioid drugs heavily for approximately more than once a week are most likely to use it daily at least for a brief period. Rapid tolerance develops to their analgesic, respiratory depression and sedative action but develops less tolerance to miotic and constipation actions.

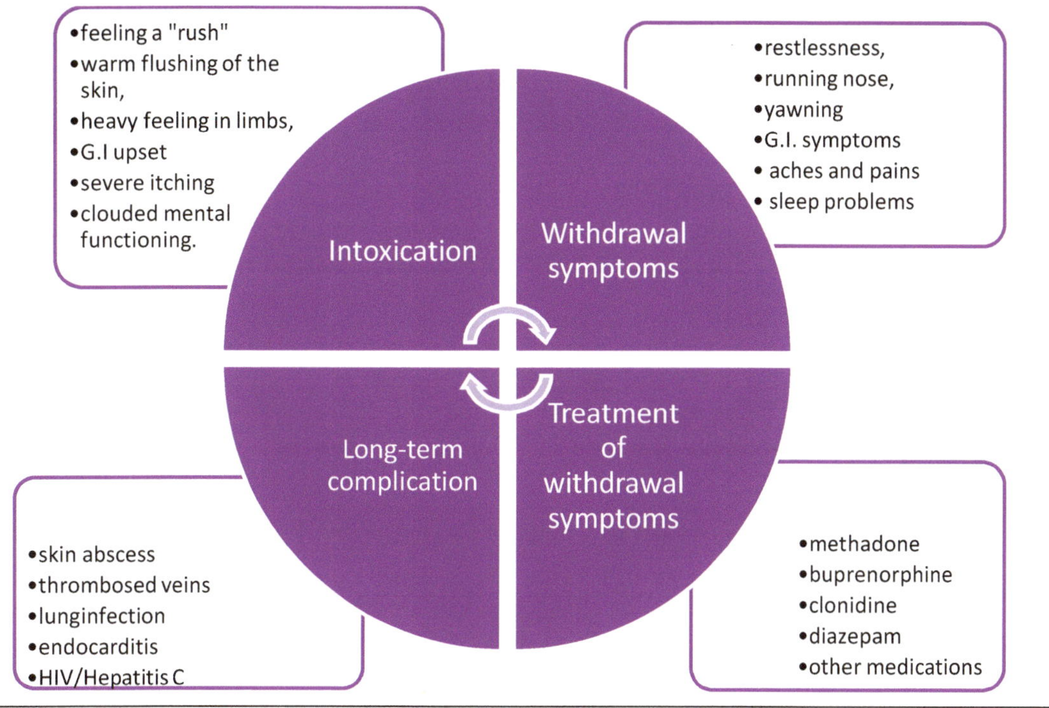

Figure 6.2.1

Long term effect

Collapsed veins (IV users), damaged nasal cartilage (snorters or sniffers), infection of the heart lining and valves, lung fibrosis, skin abscesses (swollen tissue filled with pus), skin popper (multiple craters on the skin surface), constipation, stomach cramping, sexual dysfunction (problems with orgasm, rarely impotence), depression and mania. Intravenous drug users are more prone to develop blood borne infections, such as Hepatitis B/C and HIV.

Studies have shown some loss of the brain's white matter and frontal lobe associated with chronic heroin use, which may affect decision-making, behaviour control and responses to stressful situations.

When people overdose on heroin, their breathing often slows or stops. This can decrease the amount of oxygen that reaches the brain, a condition called hypoxia. Hypoxia can have short- and long-term mental effects and effects on the nervous system, including coma and permanent brain damage.

Naloxone is a medicine that can treat an opioid overdose when it is administered immediately. It works by rapidly binding to opioid receptors and blocking the effects of heroin and other opioid drugs.

Opioid withdrawal symptoms

Withdrawal symptoms, which can begin as early as 8-12 hours after the last use of opioid for short acting preparation, such as heroin and it can be a bit prolonged for long-acting opioid preparation, such as methadone and LAAM.

Withdrawal symptoms are restlessness, lacrimation, rhinorrhoea, yawning, perspiration, G.I. symptoms, severe muscle aches, bone pain, sleep problems, low grade fever, cold flashes with goose bumps ("cold turkey"), uncontrollable leg movements ("kicking the habit") and craving.

Opioid withdrawal symptoms do not generally cause tremor, confusion, delirium or seizures, the presence of these signs should raise the possibility of comorbid alcohol or benzodiazepine dependence.

Treatment of opioid withdrawal symptoms

A wide range of medications can be used to treat opioid withdrawal symptoms, for example, methadone, buprenorphine, and clonidine. Other medications can be used for symptomatic treatment, such as loperamide (diarrhoea), NSAIDS (pain), metoclopramide (nausea), diazepam for agitation and promethazine for sleep. Buprenorphine is the best medication for opioid detoxification, which can be used as a maintenance agent.

Methadone can be a good option for those patients who want to be on opioid agonist maintenance. It is relatively a safe option for pregnant and lactating clients.

However, availability of these medications in the remote Indian communities could be a challenging issue.

Therefore, more readily available medications, such as clonidine and diazepam are the most pragmatic treatment options for opioid withdrawal in the remote Indian settings.

A study published from National Drug Dependence and Treatment Centre, AIIMS Delhi, endorsed successful use of tramadol for the management of opioid use disorders.

The American Psychiatric Association (APA) practice guidelines for substance abuse disorders recommended an initial dose of clonidine 0.1 mg PO three times (total 0.3 mg per 24 hours), which is usually enough to suppress signs of opiate withdrawal. Higher doses of clonidine which is up to 1mg/day, may be acceptable during inpatient detoxification because nursing staff can monitor hypotension and sedation. It is recommended to hold the dose of clonidine if blood pressure falls below 90/60 mmHg, resuming it again when BP returns to normal. The APA guidelines recommend limiting outpatient dispensing for unsupervised use to a 3-day supply of clonidine because treatment requires careful dose titration and clonidine overdoses can be life-threatening.

Additionally, there was a study which used quetiapine for outpatient opioid withdrawal symptoms. The dose of Quetiapine varied from 200mg to 600mg daily.

Ultrarapid detoxification

The acute phase of opioid withdrawal can be markedly shortened by using opioid antagonist to remove opioid agonist from opioid receptors. This type of detoxification can be conducted under general anaesthesia. Thus, detox phase can be shortened to a day or two.

Ear acupuncture

Acudetox is a well-established acupuncture method that targets specific points on the ear involving detox and craving pathways. It has been shown to reduce cravings for drugs, minimize withdrawal symptoms, help control agitation and anxiety, while increasing calmness, energy, concentration, and sleep.

6.3 Cocaine addiction

Cocaine is a brain stimulant substance which is made from the leaves of the coca plant. Cocaine usually looks like a fine, white, crystal powder. Drug dealers often mix it with things like corn-starch, talcum powder, flour to increase profits as well as potency. The combination of cocaine and heroin is called Speedball. Cocaine can be snorted, smoked, or injected. Cocaine crystal is heated to produce vapours that are inhaled into the lungs.

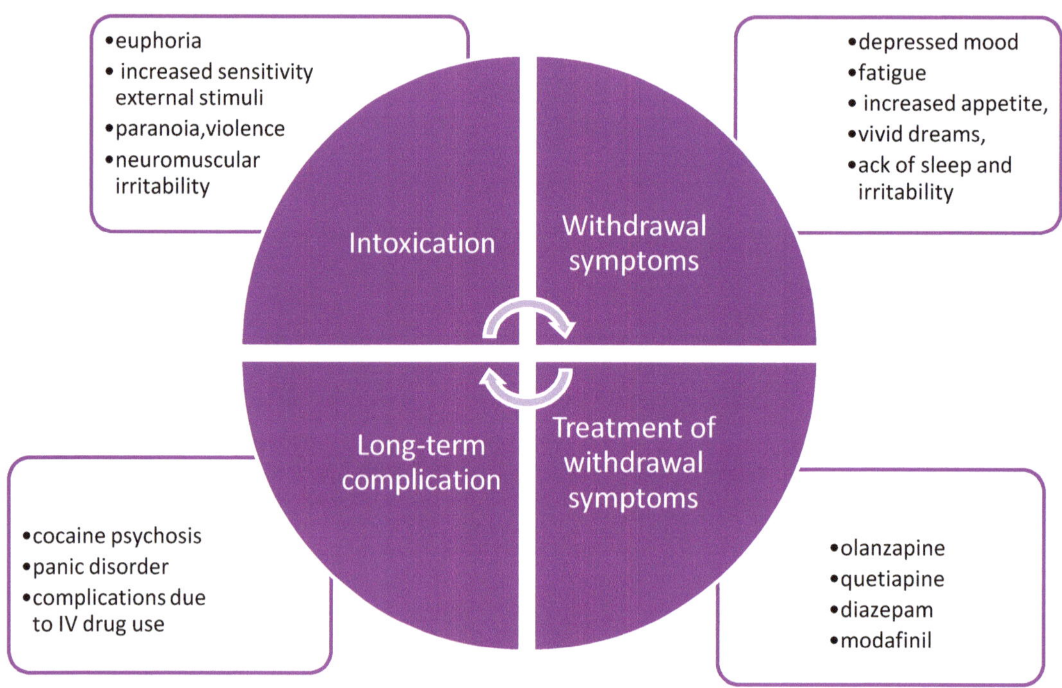

Figure 6.3.1

Serious complications due to cocaine intoxication are seizure, movement disorder, cardiac arrhythmia, stroke, and delirium.

Long-term effect

- Cocaine psychosis: People experience paranoid psychotic symptoms or tactile hallucination (cocaine bug) due to use of cocaine. Cocaine psychosis has a high propensity for relapse if they use cocaine in future due to brain sensitisation.
- Panic disorder: The brain sensitisation theory is also applicable to cocaine induced panic disorder, which may last for many months even after discontinuation of cocaine.
- Cocaine Withdrawal symptoms
- Depressed mood, fatigue, increased appetite, vivid dreams, drug craving, lack of sleep and irritability. Cocaine withdrawal phase may resemble a depressive episode.

Treatment of cocaine withdrawal symptoms

Detoxification from psychostimulants can be undertaken outside a hospital setting if the home environment is supportive and there are no stimulants or other psychoactive drugs accessible at home.

However, if the person is homeless, has a history of protracted or multiple withdrawals, is severely dependent, or has a concomitant significant medical or psychiatric illness that cannot be appropriately managed in the community, a supervised or hospital setting may be more appropriate.

Cocaine withdrawal symptoms generally recover within a few weeks. However, mood symptoms and intermittent craving may last longer for months. There is no approved medication for cocaine withdrawal symptoms. But certain medications, such as olanzapine/quetiapine and modafinil, are currently under investigation.

6.4 Amphetamine and amphetamine like substance addiction

This group of substances includes amphetamine, methamphetamine, MDMA, stimulant medications, khat (cathinone), and other substances that fall into this group, such as methcathinone, fenethylline, ephedrine, pseudoephedrine, methylphenidate and MDMA or 'Ecstasy' – an amphetamine-type derivative with hallucinogenic properties.

Mechanism of action

Releases monoamine from nerve terminals, damage to blood brain barrier, brain oedema and inflammation

Routes of use

Oral, smoking, injection, and vapour inhalation. Drug using people make different makeshift equipment to facilitate their drug using habit, which is called drug paraphernalia.

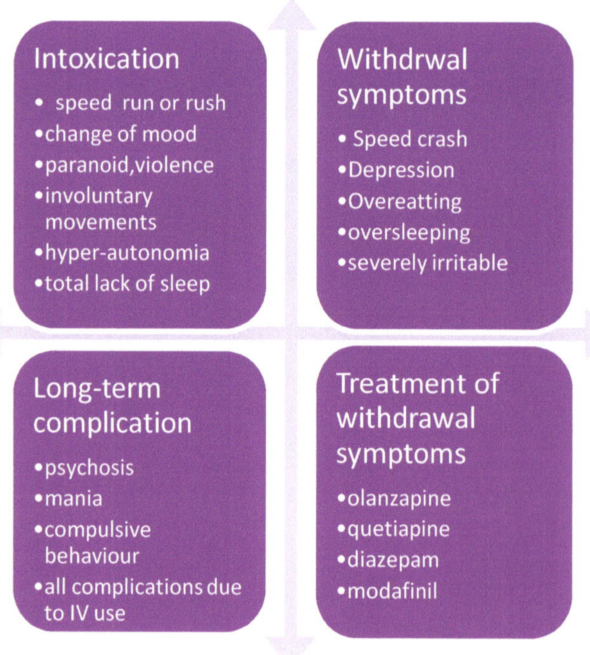

Figure 6.4.1

Signs of intoxication

Speed 'Run or Rush'

Behavioural symptoms- elevated mood, overtalkativeness, hyperactivity, irritability, aggression, bruxism, decreased sleep decreased appetite, weight loss, and paranoid behaviour.

Autonomic symptoms- high blood pressure, high pulse, increased perspiration, dilated pupil nausea, vomiting, decreased appetitive and weight loss.

Neuromuscular irritability- dystonia, dyskinesia, stereotype movements and seizure.

Signs of amphetamine withdrawal

Speed 'Crash' - oversleeping, overeating, irritability, depression, fatigue, and suicidality

Trajectory of amphetamine use- amphetamine usually runs a course characterised by few days to weeks of speed run followed by crashing, which is generally precipitated by an interruption in supply of drugs or exhaustion.

Acute Toxicity

Particularly with IV Methamphetamine use

- Cardiovascular- arrhythmia, hypertension, tachycardia, and heart attack
- Cognitive - confusion, delirium, stroke,
- Neuromuscular - seizure, come, jaw clenching, repetitive stereotyped movements, dystonia, dyskinesia, and stereotyped behaviour.
- Renal- rhabdomyolysis and acute renal failure

Comorbid mental disorder

- Onset of mental disorder, whether during intoxication or withdrawal.
- Types of psychiatric disorders- depression, mania, psychosis, panic attacks, compulsive behaviour, severe sleep disturbances, suicidality, violence, and risk-

taking behaviour (driving, unprotected sex, fight). Amphetamine increases the risk of psychosis approximately five times.

- Amphetamine induced psychosis usually lasts for weeks to months rarely extended beyond few months. It has a propensity to relapse during subsequent use of even small amphetamine due to neuronal sensitization (kindling). The diagnosis of amphetamine-induced psychosis generally comes under doubt if the duration of psychosis is more than a month, and then it is deemed an independent psychosis.

Nature of amphetamine induced psychosis.

- Paranoid delusion in 80% of cases and hallucination in 70% of cases.
- Patients usually have clear consciousness and intact reality testing.
- Presence of vivid visual or tactile hallucination in the context of amphetamine abuse will raise the possibility of drug-induced psychosis.
- Paranoid schizophrenia, if developed in the context of amphetamine use, is usually due to long term and heavy use. Amphetamine has no causal link with schizophrenia, but it can probably unmask psychosis in persons with the pre-existing vulnerability of brain.
- Patients with amphetamine-induced psychosis seem to be sensitized and will experience acute psychosis during re-exposure to small doses of amphetamine.
- Amphetamine induced psychosis is treated with atypical antipsychotics, such as olanzapine and quetiapine, for three to six months.
- Medication for amphetamine withdrawal symptoms
- No medication has been demonstrated to alleviate amphetamine withdrawal effectively, but some medications may be partially helpful.
- Mirtazapine is used for depressive symptoms which is often associated with psychotic symptoms in the context of amphetamine abuse, and the response to treatment is evident.
- Short-term use of benzodiazepines (diazepam 5 to 10mg QID) and antipsychotics (olanzapine 2.5-5mg BD) for control of irritability and agitation a maximum period of few weeks depending upon tolerability and treatment response.

- Modafinil can also be used, but it is not yet an approved medication for amphetamine withdrawal treatment.

6.5 Hallucinogen addiction

This group includes LSD, mescaline, MDMA, Psilocybin, magic mushrooms etc. They are usually used orally. The prevalence hallucinogen use in India has not been properly estimated.

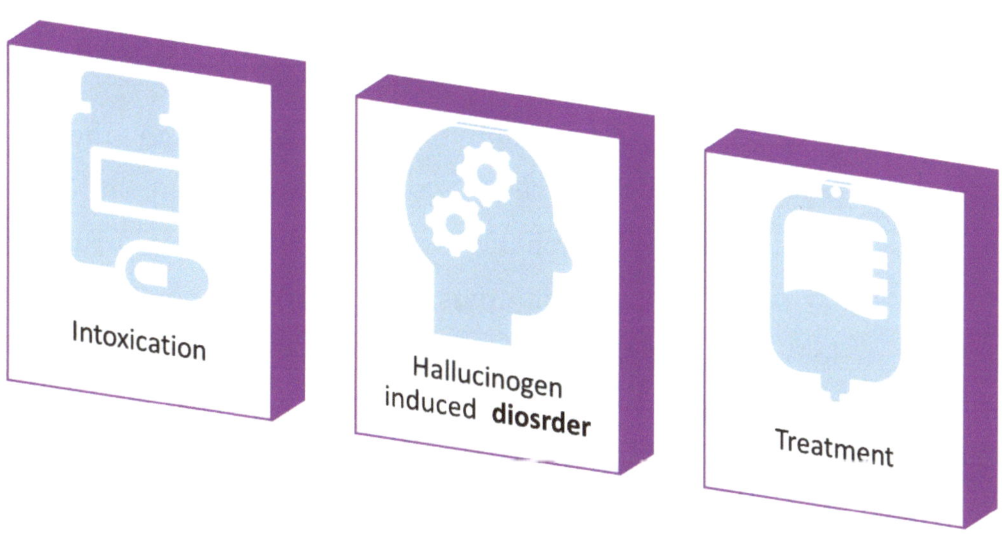

Figure 6.5.1

Hallucinogen Intoxication

- Autonomic hyper-arousal is a common occurrence.
- Psychological symptoms such as marked anxiety, panic attacks, depression, paranoid ideations, depersonalization, derealisation, illusions, and heightened sense of perception

Persistent perceptual disturbances

It can be precipitated by either prolonged use or just one-off use. Symptoms are generally precipitated after entering a dark environment. Perceptual disturbances may include geometric distortion, macropsia (objects look bigger), micropsia (object looks smaller), a false perception of movement in the peripheral field, flashes of colour, aeropsia (able to see the air). Visual symptoms that repeatedly occur after drug use, which do not last long, are called flashback or a bad trip. In most patients, their reality testing is usually preserved during flashback experiences, and hence these experiences are considered a type of pseudo-hallucination.

Treatment of hallucination induced perceptual disorder is benzodiazepine rather than antipsychotic medication.

Hallucinogen induced psychotic disorder.

The patient may experience psychotic symptoms immediately after the use of hallucinogens or after a lucid interval. If psychotic symptoms are present with impaired reality testing, a hallucinogen-induced psychotic disorder is made. Post hallucinogen psychotic symptoms may include mood symptoms, grandiosity, paranoid symptoms, multimodal hallucination, and hyper-religiosity. Individuals who have developed psychotic symptoms after one-time use of LSD without describing a typical trip are more likely to be suffering from independent rather than drug psychotic disorder. Unlike schizophrenia, the negative symptoms, prodromal phase, and impairment in interpersonal interaction are less conspicuous in hallucinogen induced psychotic disorder. Antipsychotic medications are the mainstay of treatment. Sometimes it may require other medications such as mood stabilizer, benzodiazepine, and antidepressant medication.

6.6 Inhalants addiction

Types of inhalant addiction

Inhalational substances may be of four types: aerosol, such as body spray / deodorant, volatile substances, such as paint thinners, gases (nitrous oxide), nitrites (room fresheners) and adhesives(dendrites)

Age group of the inhalant users

Adolescent age groups usually misuse inhalational drugs; adolescents diagnosed with conduct disorder usually become regular inhalants. An Indian survey reported that nearly 20% of middle school and high school children experimented with inhalational substances. Another Indian study also showed that volatile substances were the first substance misused by many chronic substance-dependent persons. Another Indian study conducted among street children in India reported that inhalant use is as high as 48%.

Inhalants are popular among adolescents due to their low price, household availability, and evasion of detection by parents and schoolteachers. It is difficult to detect the inhalant use problem unless reported by the person using it. Sometimes they may have a perioral or peri-nasal rash, or they may display unexplained intermittent behavioural changes.

Certain inhalants are linked to sudden sniffing death, due to precipitating life-threatening cardiac arrhythmia, such as butane, aerosols etc.

Detection of inhalant in urine drug screen is difficult and one need to take special precautions for that and need to repeated urine samples collected randomly and over short period.

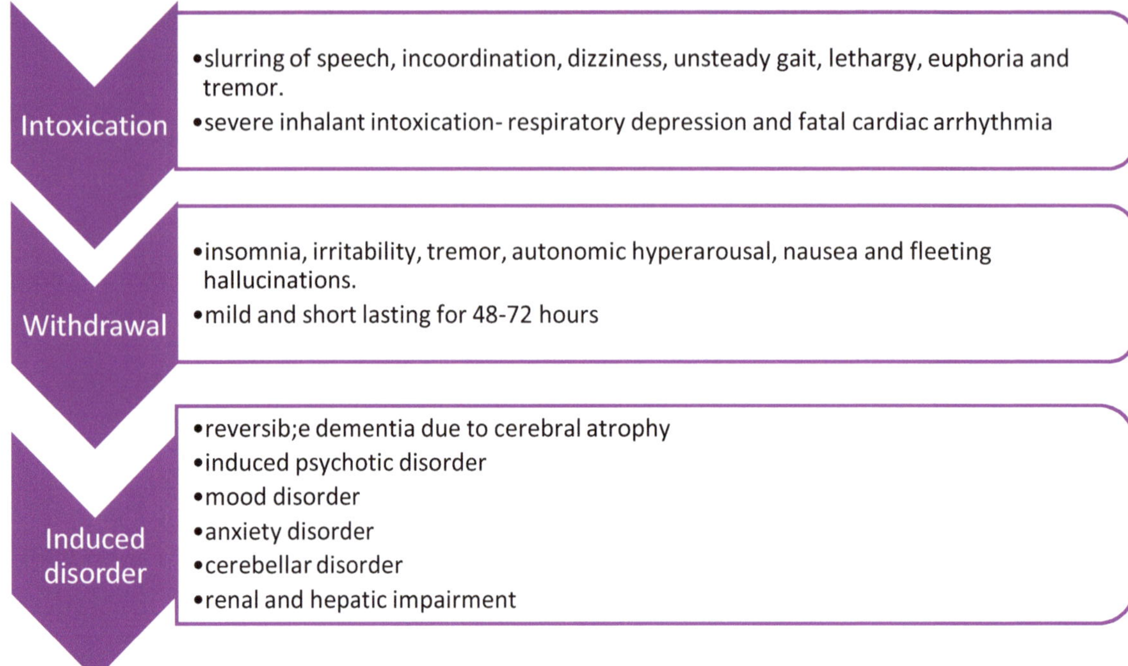

Figure 6.6.1

Long-term effect from inhalants addiction

Physical health problem

renal dysfunction, hepatic impairment, pulmonary disorders, cerebellar degeneration, cortical atrophy and even dementia.

Inhalant induced dementia

Nearly all persons who develop dementia after inhalant use are dependent on it. Alcoholism is often comorbid with inhalant use in this group and history of head injury is also very common in them. Generally, dementia is reversible after discontinuation of inhalants.

Inhalant induced psychotic disorder

Inhalant induced psychosis is usually short lasting and appears during intoxication. May need antipsychotic if causes significant disruption. Inhalant induced long-term psychosis is usually dubious.

Inhalant induced mood disorder

Depression, mania, or mixed features. Usually short lasting. Risk of self -harm and suicide is high. Seldom requires antidepressant or mood stabilizer medications.

Inhalant induced anxiety disorder

Short lasting generalized anxiety and panic attacks are most common.

Treatment of inhalant withdrawal symptoms

There is specific medication available. Benzodiazepine which is used for alcohol withdrawal is contraindicated for inhalants withdrawal despite there may be some similarities between alcohol and inhalant withdrawal symptoms. Use of benzodiazepine to counteract inhalant induced behavioural problem may result in serious complications such as respiratory depression.

6.7 Benzodiazepine addiction

Benzodiazepines are a commonly prescribed medication for sleep and anxiety. Approximately 20-30% patients with alcohol problems also abuse benzodiazepine. Many people take benzodiazepine regularly even without any prescription in India.

Mild withdrawal symptoms may occur with abrupt discontinuation of therapeutic doses after four weeks of benzodiazepine treatment. More severe withdrawal symptoms develop after 3-4 months of treatment at the therapeutic dose.

Benzodiazepine discontinuation syndrome

Any patient who has taken a benzodiazepine for longer than 3–4 weeks is likely to have discontinuation syndrome if the drug is ceased abruptly. Risk of withdrawal is greatest in patients with underlying chronic anxiety disorder or insomnia who are taking high doses of benzodiazepines over longer period.

Benzodiazepine discontinuation syndrome can be divided into three types.

Rebound symptoms are symptoms for which the benzodiazepine was originally prescribed that return in a more severe form after its discontinuation.

Recurrent symptoms mean the original symptoms return at or below the original intensity.

Withdrawal symptoms are slightly different kind of symptoms which occur following benzodiazepine discontinuation. Withdrawal symptoms are more prominent with shorter acting benzodiazepine and after rapid withdrawal. Withdrawal symptoms generally peaks 24-48 hours of benzodiazepine discontinuation for short acting ones and it may be prolonged for longer acting preparation up to two weeks.

1. Benzodiazepine withdrawal symptoms

- Mood changes – anxiety and irritability
- Neuromuscular irritability - hand tremor, tachycardia,
- Autonomic hyperarousal- elevated blood pressure, increased muscle tension, muscle hyperreflexia, and myoclonus
- Psychological symptoms- multimodal hallucination and paranoia.
- Serious complication during withdrawal - delirium and seizure

2. Benzodiazepine induced disorder

3. Benzodiazepine withdrawal delirium

- It can be indistinguishable from delirium tremens.

4. Cognitive impairment

Cognitive impairment with long-term benzodiazepine even though controversial previously, now it is well established through meta-analysis. However, a drawback for most of the studies is the small sample size. There are some reports that it is more common with short-acting benzodiazepines. Common cognitive impairments are noticed in multiple areas: visuospatial ability, information processing, verbal fluency, sustained attention, and frank amnestic disorder. Benzodiazepine induced dementia is a controversial entity.

5. Psychotic disorder

Transient psychotic symptoms, mainly multimodal hallucination can be seen following benzodiazepine withdrawal.

6. Other disorder

Benzodiazepine use has also been associated with mood disorder, anxiety, panic attacks, sleep disorder and sexual dysfunction.

7. Paradoxical reaction

Benzodiazepines are CNS depressant. Hence, they are supposed to have sedation and calming effect. However, it can rarely cause significant agitation and disinhibition, which is called a paradoxical reaction. The main features of paradoxical reaction are over talkativeness, labile emotion, psychomotor agitation, insomnia, poor sleep, aggression, hostility, and violent behaviour. The prevalence of this is less than 1%.

The cause is unclear, or it may be an idiosyncratic reaction. It is difficult to predict and diagnose this condition. It is often being misdiagnosed as psychosis. The risk factors for the paradoxical reaction are underlying structural brain defect, vulnerable personality structure which had a history of aggression, concurrent alcohol use, high dose of benzodiazepine use, short term benzodiazepine use, short-acting benzodiazepines are more likely to cause a paradoxical reaction but may be seen with other benzodiazepines as well. Oxazepam is probably the safest based on current evidence, and long-acting benzodiazepines are better.

8. Benzodiazepines equivalent dose

Benzodiazepines equivalent dose			
Name of Benzodiazepine	Half -life (hours)	Dose (mg)	Time to peak (hours)
Alprazolam	6-12	0.25	1-2
Chlordiazepoxide	100	25	1-4
Clonazepam	36	0.25	1-4
Diazepam	100	5	1-2
Lorazepam	12	1	1-4
Oxazepam	8	15	1-4
Temazepam	10	10	2-3
Nitrazepam	30	5	0.5-2
Zolpidem	6	10	1-2
Zopiclone	6	7.5	1-2

Figure 6.7.1

Benzodiazepine has large margin of safety if taken during overdose. For example, if benzodiazepine is taken as a suicide attempt even up to more than 2 gm, it will only cause mild respiratory depression. However, if benzodiazepine overdoses taken with other CNS depressant such as alcohol, it can be fatal.

Treatment of benzodiazepine dependence

- Anyone taking benzodiazepines for 2 weeks or more should be tapered from it slowly.
- There are three main strategies for benzodiazepine detoxification: 1) slow taper and 2) substitution with a long-acting benzodiazepine and 3) loading dose strategy. Another strategy is co-administering adjuvant medications.
- The patient will decide which method of detoxification they want to try. If the slow taper option is chosen, then a 10% dose reduction every week until the medication

is completely discontinued. This method may take months before complete cessation of benzodiazepine. However, this method may be problematic with short-acting benzodiazepine because of the rapid emergence of withdrawal symptoms after dose reduction.

- In contrast, switching of short-acting benzodiazepines to long-acting benzodiazepine using dose equivalence as listed in the table may be more acceptable in some cases. After 2-3 days of stabilization on the long-acting agent, reduce it by 30% in the second or third day and then 5-10% reduction every day over 2 weeks.

- If the amount of use is unknown, start with 20 mg loading dose and then continue administering it as 10mg every hourly until mild sedation occurs.

- In terms of tapering of benzodiazepine, clinicians should be flexible about the rate of taper and let the patient decide how quickly or slowly they would like to taper off diazepam.

- Withdrawal symptoms appear earlier for drugs with short half-lives. In some cases, taking high doses of a benzodiazepine for a year or more may require several months to stop it.

- Adjuvant medications are mainly valproate and carbamazepine. Initially Carbamazepine 200-400mg BD or valproate 500 mg BD is administered. Then benzodiazepine tapering is started. By this method, faster tapering is possible, and the risk of withdrawal seizure will be less. After that, carbamazepine or valproate should be tapered off quickly over 2-4 weeks. Gabapentin, propranolol, and clonidine also can be used, but these medications will only take care of autonomic/anxiety symptoms.

- Long-term follow-up studies suggested that most patients can successfully come off benzodiazepine after multiple abstinence attempts. Some patients had a recurrence of anxiety symptoms which required psychological treatment or alternative medication options. A tiny proportion of people required recommencement of benzodiazepines.

Benzodiazepine detoxification in the context of poly-substance abuse

Benzodiazepine use is often co-morbid with other substances, particularly alcohol, opioid, and stimulants. Alcohol and benzodiazepine withdrawal require a similar type of treatment, i.e., long-acting benzodiazepines. However, in the co-morbidity with the opioid, benzodiazepine should be detoxified first and then opioid. This is because the combination of benzodiazepine with opioid agonist treatment such as Methadone can cause fatal respiratory failure. Like alcohol, benzodiazepine and stimulant withdrawal can be dealt with simultaneously.

6.8 Nicotine addiction

Nicotine use is the most used substance. Nicotine use is highly prevalent in the psychiatric population (80%). Nicotine is a cytochrome enzyme inducer. Smoking cessation can increase the blood level of different medications. Nicotinic-cholinergic receptors lie on dopamine neurons. Hence nicotine increases dopamine. Nicotine also increases epinephrine, norepinephrine, and serotonin in the brain.

Age of onset of nicotine use is adolescence. Nicotine use usually starts at a young age due to peer pressure. Other high-risk groups who have a high propensity for nicotine use are adolescents with low academic performance, adolescents with conduct problems, depression, and low self-esteem. Nicotine is a gateway drug, which means that it often leads to using other hard drugs, such as cannabis and amphetamine, in children's problematic group.

Nicotine withdrawal symptoms

- Nicotine withdrawal syndrome starts within 24 hours of cessation and lasts for 3-4 weeks.
- Common features of nicotine withdrawal are irritable mood, insomnia, anxiety, difficulty concentrating, restlessness, craving, decreased heart rate, increased appetite and weight gain.
- Nicotine withdrawal symptoms can often be misconstrued as psychotic agitation or agitated depression in the context of underlying psychiatric problems.

- Nicotine withdrawal may cause a relapse of psychotic symptoms and temporarily worsen self-harm thoughts and aggressive behaviour in the psychiatric setting.
- Fagerstrom Questionnaire is an evidence-based instrument, which is used to assess the extent and severity of nicotine dependence.
- The severity indicators of nicotine dependence are:
  - time to first smoke, 2) total number of smokes per day, and 3) tendency to continue smoking despite having significant health complications secondary to nicotine use.

Treatment of nicotine dependence

5-10% of self-quitters are successful on one attempt and 50% may be able to give up after repeated attempts.

Readiness to change assessment is essential initial step, which is usually assessed by a standard Readiness to Change Questionnaire.

If an individual is prepared to give up cigarette, it is expected to set a quit date. Some people may prefer abrupt cessation on the quit date, but others may want to cut it down whilst taking NRT at the same time.

Strategies management for nicotine withdrawal

Nicotine replacement therapy (NRT) can be offered in various forms, such as gums, lozenges, inhaler, and patch. Additionally, some medications are used for this purpose, such as bupropion, varenicline, and nortriptyline. If the person is not allergic to NRT and is willing to take it, it is prudent to start with nicotine patch supplemented by gums, lozenges, nasal spray, or inhaler. Nicotine patch has three common strengths: 21 mg /24 hours, 14mg/24 hours and 7 mg/24 hours. 7mg/24 hours patch is rarely used. The 21mg/24 hours is most commonly used. Mild smokers may need 14 mg/24 hours patch. The commonest side effect of nicotine patch is rash. The patch must be taken out at night before going to bed. Both gums and lozenges come as 1 mg and 2 mg strengths, the bigger one is used for heavy smokers (> 10 cigarettes a day. The drawback of gums and lozenges is bad taste and decreased appetite. Many people prefer inhalers due to their resemblance to cigarettes, and they are better tolerated. Additionally, Bupropion can be used in those cases where nicotine dependence is comorbid with depression. The most serious drawbacks of bupropion are side effects such as the emergence of psychosis and precipitation of seizure. The dose of bupropion is 150mg BD initially and then 300 mg BD. Furthermore, varenicline is a partial agonist of the nicotine receptor, which many nicotine-dependent persons prefer because of its convenience in tablet form. However, the major drawback of varenicline is that it can negatively impact on mental health. For example, it can precipitate psychotic symptoms and can make depressed patients suicidal and agitated. It can also interfere with sleep. The varenicline dose is 0.5 mg mane (first three days), gradually increased to 0.5 mg BD (4-7 days) and then 1 mg BD. More recently, E-cigarette has become quite popular. E-cigarettes are operated by battery, and they have a close resemblance to original cigarettes. It is also called vaping because it releases smokes on exhalation. E-cigarettes usually contain nicotine in a relatively small amount; E-cigarettes are devoid of other harmful substances, such as tar. The safety profile of e-cigarettes is still under investigation.

Psychological treatment

Success rate of nicotine treatment is 50% or less if treated with pharmacotherapy alone. Adjuvant psychological treatment is as important as others.

Cognitive and behavioural techniques are evidence-based treatment for nicotine addiction. Some of the basic strategies are 1) Do not keep cigarette at home,2) rapid smoking (smokes continuously up to the point of feeling nausea),3) changing environment to get rid of all triggers and 4) changing lifestyle such as meditation, stress management, physical exercise and developing alternative interests to fill in the free time.

6.9 Caffeine addiction

History of caffeine use is unknowingly missed out during substance use interview. Many people drink a large amount of caffeine every day. Caffeine may be used in hot drinks, caffeinated drinks (soft drink) and less commonly in solid form. Excessive caffeine use may cause exacerbation of underlying anxiety symptoms, precipitate panic attacks, sleep problems, and cause significant psychomotor agitation.

Intoxication of caffeine

Caffeine intoxication can be precipitated by caffeine consumption over 250 mg, more than 2-3 cups of brewed coffee in quick succession. The common clinical features of caffeine intoxication are autonomic arousal, agitation, anxiety, headache, sleep problems, gastrointestinal disturbances, tachycardia, and cardiac arrhythmia. Caffeine has a relatively short half-life. Hence caffeine intoxication resolves spontaneously.

Caffeine induced anxiety disorder.

Caffeine induced anxiety disorder can be mainly panic disorder and generalised anxiety disorder. Caffeine can also cause exacerbation of all underlying anxiety disorders. Some people with anxiety disorder have a low tolerance for caffeine and experience a great deal of anxiety after caffeine consumption.

Caffeine induced sleep disorder.

A caffeine-induced sleep disorder can be insomnia, parasomnia, hypersomnia etc.; insomnia is the most common symptom of caffeine intoxication.

Caffeine withdrawal symptoms

Caffeine withdrawal and dependence remains a controversial issue. Abrupt caffeine withdrawal may result in headache, fatigue, irritability, muscle twitching, anxiety and depression, nausea, and vomiting. Headache is the most common withdrawal symptom. It is usually short-lasting for 2-4 days.

Treatment of caffeine withdrawal

There is no specific treatment for caffeine problem. Common strategies are self-monitoring by maintaining a daily diary about caffeine use, gradual tapering of daily dose and positive reinforcement for decreasing dose.

6.10 Alcohol addiction

The lifetime risk for alcohol dependence is 10% for men and 5% in women. The age of onset of alcohol use is usually late teenage which usually becomes a dependent drinking pattern after 10 years of regular drinking. Women usually start drinking alcohol relatively later, but they progress to dependent drinking more rapidly than men. Dependent alcoholics generally go through a cycle, which starts with drinking periods followed by controlled drinking or temporary cessation followed by an escalation of alcohol intake again. The life span of an alcoholic is unfortunately shortened by 10-15 years. Patient with less severe alcohol use may achieve total abstinence; however, persons, who fulfil the criteria of alcohol dependence, are unlikely to achieve long-term abstinence without intensive treatment and support.

Alcohol intoxication

The severity of alcohol withdrawal symptoms will be dependent on the level of alcohol in their system in conjunction with their pharmacodynamic tolerance.

 For instance,

• If blood alcohol level is less than 80mg/dL, it slows motor functioning and cognitive slowing is observed.

• From 80mg to 200 mg/dL, incoordination and impaired judgement is noticed. If the level surpasses that, a range of neurological signs are noticed including alcohol blackout.

• People may even die from alcohol toxicity if blood alcohol level is more than 300mg/dL

Alcohol withdrawal symptoms

Patients are more likely to develop alcohol withdrawal if:

1. Their average daily alcohol consumption is more than 80g/day.

2. They have history of alcohol withdrawal syndrome.

3. They have scored 2 or more in CAGE questionnaire.

4. Their blood alcohol level is more than 0.15 g/100ml during initial assessment.

- **Common withdrawal symptoms**

  Mild tremor, increased perspiration, tachycardia, insomnia, nausea, and vomiting. It begins within 8 hours of abstinence, reaches the peak in a day or two, and then it is significantly diminished by the fourth or fifth day. Protracted withdrawal symptoms may last for weeks to months. Benzodiazepine is the medication of choice for alcohol withdrawal syndrome.

- **Complicated withdrawal symptoms**

  Grand mal seizure (rum fits), delirium tremens and transient hallucination
  Delirium tremens - It usually occurs after 72 hours of withdrawal and characterised by disorientation, clouding of consciousness, coarse tremor instead of fine tremor in normal withdrawal and perceptual disturbances, such as vivid visual and auditory hallucination of insects/animals. This is a medical emergency and often requires hospitalisation. The mortality rate of DT is 10-15% if it is not treated urgently. Benzodiazepine is the mainstay of treatment. General medical measures include correcting dehydration, vitamin supplementation and admitting the patient in the high dependency unit to ensure low stimulation environment and supportive care. Atypical antipsychotic can be used as a last resort to contain agitation.

- **Alcohol withdrawal seizure**

  Alcohol withdrawal seizure usually takes place after 48-72 hours of abstinence. It is a grand mal type of seizure. The usual pattern is multiple seizures in a quick succession approximately 48 hours after the last drink. EEG tracing is usually normal. Withdrawal seizure can lead to delirium tremens in 30% of cases. The treatment of alcohol withdrawal seizure is benzodiazepine rather than antiepileptic medications. In patients with a prior seizure history or severe alcohol withdrawal, diazepam loading is recommended. Carbamazepine effectively prevents alcohol withdrawal seizures but is not as effective as a benzodiazepine. The patient should be admitted into the hospital for the assessment of other causes of seizures.

- **Wernicke encephalopathy**

  It is an acute neuropsychiatric disorder precipitated by the sudden withdrawal of alcohol from the system. Wernicke encephalopathy (WE) involve periventricular and mammillary bodies micro-haemorrhages, and Korsakoff psychosis involves necrosis of thalamic nucleus and maxillary bodies. WE are characterised by a triad of confusion, ataxia and ophthalmoplegia (lateral rectus muscle weakness). This condition is due to thiamine deficiency. It can be potentially life-threatening if it is not diagnosed and treated early with thiamine supplementation. Thiamine needs to be administered with 500 mg intravenously 3 times a day for 2-3 days. After that, oral thiamine (300mg daily) should be continued until symptoms persist. If thiamine is prescribed as a prophylactic agent, it should be prescribed in a dose of 200mg per day for three months after abstinence from alcohol (South Australia Drug and Alcohol Service). During the acute phase of treatment of WE, it is important to administer thiamine before administration of glucose to prevent worsening of encephalopathy as thiamine is a cofactor in the metabolism of glucose.

- **Korsakoff's psychosis**

  Psychosis is a misnomer here. It is characterised by mainly anterograde and to some extent retrograde memory loss. It is preceded by Wernicke encephalopathy, which is often being unrecognised. As many as 2 out of 3 WE patients if untreated may turn into Korsakoff's psychosis. Other associated features of KS are confabulation (unconsciously substituting gaps in the recent memory with past or false memory), apathy (lack of emotional reactivity) and peripheral neuropathy.

KS often leads to a permanent condition. 1 in 3 patients of KS may improve partially with long-term use of thiamine (100-200mg) orally for several months. Pyridoxine may help with peripheral neuropathy.

Long-term complication

1. Alcohol-induced dementia

Long-term alcohol use may cause impairment in executive function, memory, information processing and intellectual functioning. Some signs of cerebral atrophy are evident in 50-70% of patients. There are several reasons for alcohol-induced dementia, such as head trauma, the direct toxic effect of alcohol and vitamin deficiencies. The brain changes can be reversed after achieving total abstinence for a sustained period.

2. Alcohol induced depression

5-10% of chronic alcohol users may report moderate to severe depressive symptoms even after abstaining from alcohol for four weeks or more. In this case, they can be labelled as an independent depressive disorder. However, it is not uncommon to feel depressed during the withdrawal phase of alcohol. Some low-grade mood changes persist for months, which is generally considered a normal course of withdrawal symptoms.

3. Alcohol induced anxiety disorder

Anxiety symptoms are common in the context of acute as well as protracted withdrawal state. Panic disorder and social phobia more commonly present with alcohol use disorder. Prolonged abstinence from alcohol generally helps with reduction of anxiety symptoms.

4. Alcohol induced psychotic disorder

A small proportion of patients (3%) reports psychotic symptoms in the context of heavy use or withdrawal. Some psychotic symptoms may persist even when they are not drinking. Psychotic symptoms may consist of delusion and hallucinations. Visual hallucinations are commonly reported during the withdrawal phase, which includes bugs crawling on the wall. Auditory hallucinations are often voicing that is usually frightening and paranoid in nature. Visual and auditory hallucinations may occur simultaneously.

Hallucinations occur on the background of clear sensorium in contrast with the clouded consciousness characteristic of alcohol withdrawal delirium. Antipsychotic medication should not be used in isolation (i.e., without adequate benzodiazepine cover). They do not adequately prevent the onset of alcohol withdrawal delirium and may lower the seizure threshold. Antipsychotic medications, such as olanzapine, quetiapine, risperidone is usually prescribed alcoholic hallucinosis which occurs in the context of ongoing alcohol use.

5. Comorbidity with a pre-existing psychiatric disorder

Various psychiatric illnesses may precede alcohol use problems. Antisocial personality disorder, bipolar disorder, social anxiety disorder and schizophrenia may pre-exist before commencement of alcohol. It can be postulated that alcohol drinking started as a coping mechanism in all these conditions to deal with symptoms of mental illnesses.

6. Alcoholic hallucinosis

Chronic alcohol use can result in an organic psychotic disorder, most commonly with hallucination (alcoholic hallucinosis). It can be difficult to differentiate from other causes of psychosis, such as paranoid schizophrenia. Hallucinations (usually auditory) occur whilst patients are drinking, although may persist during withdrawal, and can be mistaken for alcohol withdrawal hallucinations.

Treatment with antipsychotic medications is recommended until long-term abstinence is achieved, and symptoms ameliorate. The prognosis is usually good if long-term abstinence is maintained, although a minority (10-20%) will develop a chronic psychosis. Sodium valproate can also reduce auditory hallucinations in patients with alcoholic hallucinosis.

Biological markers for alcohol use

Biological markers reflect severity of alcohol use, even though these markers van be deranged in other conditions as well.

Gamma glutamyl transferase (GGT) - 60-70% sensitive and specific. This enzyme returns to normal within four weeks of abstinence.

Carbohydrate-deficient transferrin (CDT) - 65-80% sensitivity and specificity. It is an indicator of heavy alcohol use. It has shortest biological half-life and its level come back to normal within two weeks of abstinence.

Mean corpuscular volume (MCV) - 70% sensitive and specific. It takes up to 4 months of abstinence before returning to normal level.

Additionally, AST, ALT, uric acid, and triglycerides may also increase due heavy and long-term drinking habit.

Treatment of alcohol withdrawal symptoms

There are three medication strategies for the treatment of alcohol withdrawal symptoms:

- **Symptom triggered approach**

It involves using benzodiazepine as if required basis medication guided by alcohol withdrawal scale score. This approach is suitable for mild to moderate withdrawal symptoms.

- **Fixed dose regime**

Diazepam 20mg -80 mg in divided dosage. This approach is particularly useful for community detoxification.

- **Loading dose strategy**

This approach is most useful for complicated withdrawal symptoms (10-20 mg initially and 10mg every hourly until mild sedation occurs).

- **Ear acupuncture**

Acudetox is a well-established method of acupuncture that targets specific points on the ear which eventually influences the detoxification and craving pathways. It has been shown to reduce cravings of substances, minimize withdrawal symptoms, control agitation and anxiety, while instilling a sense of calmness, improving concentration, and promoting sleep.

Other medications for alcohol withdrawal symptoms

Carbamazepine is a safe alternative to benzodiazepines, but it is usually is not recommended for use as the first line of treatment because it has significant side effects and may not prevent secondary seizures. Topiramate is an antiepileptic. It has been proven to be partially effective to ameliorate of alcohol withdrawal symptoms. Gabapentin is well tolerated and is found to be clinically equally efficacious to lorazepam in reducing alcohol withdrawal symptoms, especially at the higher dosage dose. Antipsychotic medications can be used in conjunction with benzodiazepines to treat hallucinations or agitation in patients who do not respond well to benzodiazepines alone. Baclofen, which is a muscle relaxant, has been successfully trilled for alcohol withdrawal.

7.0 Strategies for prevention and management of alcohol use in low resource setting in the rural India

7.1 Debate of Policy Options

Throughout the world, there are different policies for alcohol and drug use. The variation of systems depends on the choices of underpinning principles adopted by the different jurisdiction. The policy viewpoints are often debatable among citizens, researchers, and government. Hence, it essential to understand the key assumptions around the dilemmas of the policy framework.

Assumption of war on substance abuse

The term was in the limelight due to President Richard Nixon's famous speech in 1971 where assumption underpinned was zero tolerance towards the illicit drug. These assumptions fuelled by the moral principles that people who consume drugs are criminal

and the banning of drugs can solve the issue. However, harsh laws created a flourishing black market in the country and an exponential increment in the prison population.

Assumption of Harm minimisation and Decriminalisation

In Australia, harm minimisation concept becomes the pivotal strategy for national drug strategy. Instead of the total banning of drugs, the focus was on reducing the harm caused by the drugs. These approaches consider deep-rooted social factors such as homelessness and unemployment and biological factors such as genetics and dependence as the cause of the problem, instead of blaming the victim for making bad choices.

Another country of interest is Portugal, where policy revolves around decriminalisation for personal use drug. Here, it is important to note that decriminalisation does not support the legalisation of drugs. It assumes that people who consume drugs should not be penalised instead of referred to the support and treatment centre.

How fund works for policy choices?

In an ideal situation, policy money should be invested for upliftment of society. While choosing a zero-tolerance policy, most funds shifted towards law enforcement agency such as police and judicial system. However, decriminalisation invests most on the prevention and treatment of drug use; hence, there is evidence of the enormous success of Portugal policy.

7.2 What approach is suitable for low resource setting of India?

The strategy may vary depending upon India's geographical regions. In many rural and remote communities in India, there are issues of availability and accessibility addiction services. For instance, substance use treatment centres are available in the metro city; however, small states but high prevalence state such as Tripura still lacks addiction treatment services. Another key point to note in the current policy for substance use in India gives overemphasis on law enforcement activities. Although India sanctioned illicit drugs in the NDPS Act 1985, the strategy remains ineffective in controlling drug menace.

For a small community of Tripura region, the cultural factors play an important role while considering policy strategy. Tagging young adults as criminals would not work effectively for drug addiction as an individual would feel more isolated from society. Hence, tailored harm minimisation strategies would be effective for alcohol and drug use in Tripura.

7.3 How Drug policy is different from other health policies?

Traditionally, health policy comprises law, regulation, and funds utilised to treat and prevent disease. But drug policy is much more complicated than other health policies. There are many other factors which may potentially impact development and implementation of the drug policy, such as social factors (societal attitude and norms), drug problem (overdose, criminality, and accidents), and other social policies (state welfare scheme).

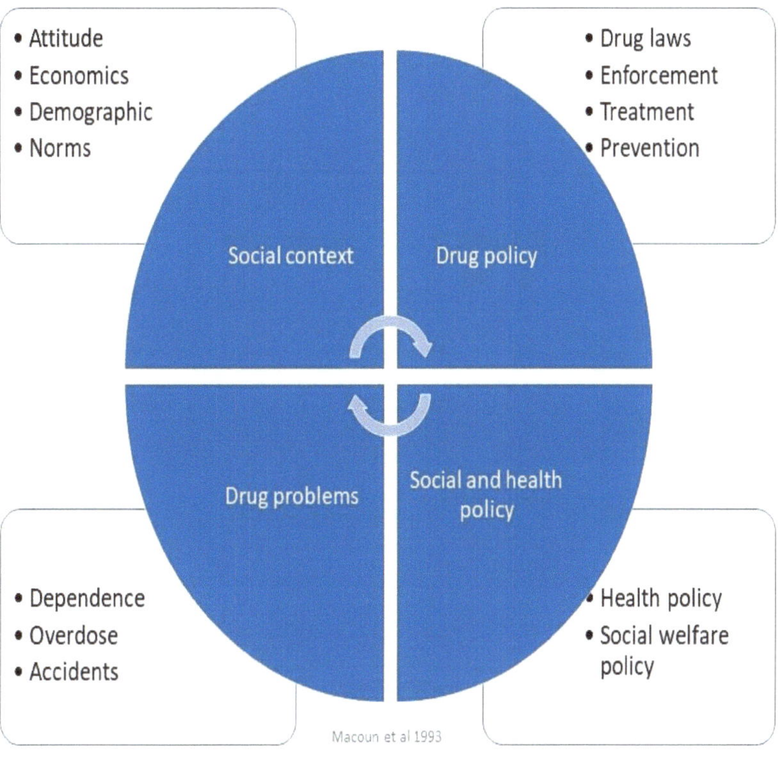

Figure 7.3.1

One example of how social factors influence drug policy is the use of cannabis in India. The use of cannabis in India dates back to thousands of years ago. The ancient Ayurvedic System of India used cannabis for the treatment of several health conditions. The name of cannabis was also being mentioned in Hindu mythology. There are three types of cannabis available in India, such as Bhang (derived from leaves of Cannabis Sativa), Ganja (derived from flower tops of Cannabis Sativa) and Charas (derived from resinous exudates of Cannabis Sativa). When National Drugs and Psychotropic Substances Act (NDPS) was enforced in 1985 in India, the illegalisation of cannabis was vehemently argued because of it is being a culturally sanctioned substance in some parts of India. As a result, Bhang was excluded from the NDPS Act, and it was socially sanctioned for use in various cultural and religious festivals. However, Ganja and Charas were enlisted under the NDPS Act. In contrast, the use of any cannabis products is banned in most countries, and the defaulters are subjected to serious legal consequences, including imprisonment and corporal punishment.

7.4 Do social attitude and opinion significantly impact drug policy of a country?

One example of how drug factors influence drug policy is increasing drug cost due to a reduction in drugs supply through law enforcement and black marketing. People may indulge in various antisocial activities to meet up the higher cost of drugs. The only way to prevent it is by supplying the legal medications through clinics to close the gap between availability and demands for drugs. Another example of drug factor is accidental overdose on the addictive drugs, such as opioids. Thus, drug policy should address how to manage overdose risk in the local region, such as supplying naloxone injection and setting up medically supervised injection rooms.

One example of how social policy is the impacts of the social welfare scheme on drug use. More recently, Australia is thinking about mandatory drug testing for people receiving social welfare payments. If they become positive on illicit drugs during random testing, the government is thinking about restricting their social welfare payment. This approach's problem is that drug addiction is an illness, and coercive approach will be unlikely successful in achieving long-term abstinence.

7.5 How does the view of society about drug use impact the policy?

World Health Organisation (1969) defines "a drug as any substance except for food and water, which when taken into the body, alters its function, physically and/or psychologically." Considering this definition, drug use is not at all an uncommon situation in our society. The history of drug use dates back to thousands of years ago. There is no society in the world which has not used some form of drugs. Many people drink tea or coffee, but they do not consider them as drugs because they are socially approved substances. Similarly, opium is a culturally sanctioned drugs in some rural Indian communities. While possession of alcohol is a punishable offence in Saudi Arabia, it is being rampantly used in most countries. When alcohol is banned in the USA for almost a decade, it caused more problems than benefits due to rampant black marketing, increased organised crimes, and significant government revenue losses. A similar type of experiment of banning of alcohol also failed in the Indian state of Kerala. Thus, views of society about drug use may differ, and we all use some forms of drugs in one way or another.

7.6 Is total drug-free state an unrealistic option?

Most of the drug policies focus on total abstinence and drug-free country. It is usually not acknowledged by them that there will always be some people who use drugs. Thus, it is essential to include some harm reduction strategies and policy. As many people die of opioid overdose, some measures need to be taken to prevent the disastrous outcome. When conventional drugs, such as heroin is not available in the market due to stricter law enforcement, people may turn into cheaper and easily available counterfeit options, such as carfentanil which is sold as heroin by the drug dealer. Cafentanil is a veterinary sedative medication, frequently used on the animals. It is a relatively cheaper medication. Hence, it is preferred by the drug dealers. However, this cheaper option may turn out to be much more powerful and toxic. As a result, so-called heroin users might accidentally overdose on carfentanil. Similarly, the risk of spread of HIV/Hepatitis C may exponentially increase in the injectable drug users. This group of patients avoid seeking help due to fear of serious legal consequences. Thus, the policy shift from a very punitive approach to inclusive public approach is required. If society can normalise drug use behaviour and integrate drug users into the mainstream society, it will automatically reduce overall drug use, fatality due to overdose and black marketing. Punitive measures cause social isolation of substances users as well.

7.7 How does drug decriminalisation work?

Portugal is leading the way to the drug decriminalisation policy. This policy endorses taking out the bulk of drug funds from supply reduction activities and investing it in reconnecting drug-using people in the society. This policy has no mercy for drug producers or drug dealers, but it intends to show a more humane approach towards people who possess drugs for their personal use. This policy aims to invest money for job creation and recovery-oriented activities for drug users. These activities may help people to rediscover purpose in your life and reconnect them with the broader society.

7.8 Why drafting of a drug policy is a difficult affair?

The excise revenue on alcohol significantly contributes to the total revenue of the country across the world. For instance, some Indian states are increasingly dependent on the drug revenue to pay their bills, which may go up to 20% of the total revenue. In many Indian states, excise revenue on alcohol remains the second or third highest contributor to its total revenue. If you add up tobacco tax revenue, tobacco with alcohol will contribute to at least one-third of the state total revenue. Thus, any reduction or banning of alcohol causes significant revenue loss for the state, impacting state's expenditure in many important social areas.

Additionally, the legal status of the drug may vary a lot in society. Some drug may be banned today, which was permissible yesterday. Some society may approve some drugs for the religious sacrament, but the same drug may be banned in other places. There may be some stereotype related to drugs and drug use, which may get in the way of an objective assessment of drug use and drug related harms. Drug policies are usually developed based on some anecdotal evidence or in the aftermath of some critical incident. Judgement about drugs is often formed following someone experience with the drug or experience of someone else they know. For instance, some people who use drugs to socialise with their peer group may interpret drug use as a good thing. On the other hand, those who have experienced road traffic accidents, domestic violence or health problems may interpret drug use is a bad thing. The policymakers and lawmakers personal experience may influence the making of the drug policy. Thus, it is essential to form an objective perspective about drugs and drug use rather than forming an opinion based on anecdotes and myths.

7.9 Importance of evidence for drafting a drug policy

Everyone has an opinion about drugs and drug use, as if the drug use issue is everyone's business. Any discussion about this issue usually generates a conflict of opinion between different members of society. Some people may form an opinion based on their personal knowledge and experience. Other people may form their opinion about drugs by gathering information from the websites. Some people may make an opinion about drugs and drug use from an isolated incident or some anecdotal evidence. Before developing a drug policy, it is important to extract evidence from various reliable scientific publication and evidence-based facts rather than public opinions and anecdotal evidence.

7.10 Summary of complexities around formulation of the drug policy

The drug policy is a much more complex issue. It goes far beyond law enforcement, regulation, treatment, and substance use disorder prevention. Many other social, clinical, and political factors potentially influence the National drug policy's successful implementation. While overreliance on the supply reduction issues may cause more harm than benefit, simultaneous implementation of harm reduction strategies may narrow the gap between different harm minimisation strategies.

8.0 Harm Minimisation Strategy

Harm minimisation is an overarching term which consists of three pillars of demand reduction, supply reduction and harm reduction. Harm minimisation approach aims at reducing the harm associated with substance use through the coordinated and multiagency approach. All those pillars should be given equal importance while developing the policy. One of the critical reasons for the failure of harm minimisation is emphasising on one pillar and neglecting the other two. For instance, supply reduction encompasses law enforcement, and policymakers tend to incline towards the legislator approach and ignoring demand reduction and harm reduction, which involves early intervention and creating a support system for addiction.

8.1 How do you know whether a drug policy working or not?

- Reduction of recent use (over last 12 months) of substance
- Reduction of arrests due to substance-related offence
- Reduction of the number of victims due to drug-related incidents
- Reduction of the substance-related burden of disease
- Reduction in the number of substance-related mortality

8.2 Demand Reduction

Demand reduction aims at reducing the public desire for legal as well as illegal substances. It aims to prevent or delay substance use uptake, reducing misuse and supporting individual from drug dependence issues. This strategy aims at delaying the onset of use and public demands for substance. This strategy also supports people to reduce or discontinue use of substance through evident-based treatment strategies.

To achieve this objective, health provider leadership's role provides a useful tool to build an awareness programme and put the priority of brief intervention in a primary care setting. Another suggested initiative is establishing local addiction treatment centres and support for recovering addicts, such as peer-based community support and various rehabilitative activities: life skill training and employment opportunities for recovering addicts through rehabilitation.

Strategies:

1. Price control

•Higher tax for legal substances, such as tobacco and alcohol.

Minimum floor pricing per standard drink below which alcohol cannot be sold. This strategy will reduce amount of drinking in the heavy drinkers because they prefer cheap alcohol and drink more if price of alcohol is low.

•For illicit drugs, influencing market price of illicit drugs through law enforcement and controlling the border.

2. Building community awareness and acceptance

•Targeted social marketing campaign.

•Encouraging community awareness program.

•School-based program, and high-risk group (children of substance user) program.

•Increased involvement in the community activities, such as education, cultural events, and sporting events for to raise awareness about drug use.

•Family support program to make them aware of harmful effect of drugs and building up their resilience.

•Adolescent specific program to make them aware and resilient.

•Building peer support network in the local community.

3. Restriction of promotion

•Banning advertisement

•Banning retail display

•Regulate promotion in key areas, such as those targeting young population.

•Enforcing advertising standards

4. Treatment

•Developing detoxification and rehabilitation centres in the remote community.

•Developing tailored treatment guidelines for evidence-based practice.

5. Diversion

•Diversion of clients from the legal system to treatment services.

•Enforcing drug decriminalisation policy to divert focus from the legal system to treatment services.

6. Workforce

•Building a local workforce and upskilling of local doctors in assessment of substance use disorder and brief intervention.

•Developing a network of local doctors for responsible prescription and local pharmacies for responsible dispensing.

7. Addressing social determinants

•Dealing with homelessness.

•Intervention for social isolation.

•Family support program for enabling behaviour and high expressed emotion

All demand reduction strategies mentioned above are evidence-based, but some of them may not be relevant for development of drug policy for the remote region. However, the strategies mentioned below will be more specific to the remote and low resource setting regions of the developing countries. We can call them novel strategies.

Novel Demand Reduction Strategies for the low resource setting regions

•Creating some dedicated places in the community for alcohol use so that restricted amount of alcohol can be served there.

•Restricting weekly or daily amount(rationing) of take away alcohol from the shops.

•Collaboration with alcohol producing companies for producing low-cost alcohol by using Mohammad Yunus Social Business Model (Corporate Social Responsibility).

•Developing addiction smart community by educating and empowering people from the community so that they can embrace recovering addicts and actively take part in their recovery.

8.3 Supply Reduction

Supply reduction means entails formulating strategies to monitor and disrupt production and supply of legal and illegal drugs. This strategy not only reduces local production of substances, but it also disrupts illegal importation through strict border control measures.

Strategies:

1. **Regulating production and distribution**

•Regulating production of alcohol.

•Dismantling illegally produced products.

•Dismantling criminal groups involved in the organised crime.

•Confiscation of assets derived from illicit drug activities.

2. **Regulating retail sale**

•Regulating retail licensing.

•Destroying sales of illegal products.

•Regulating trading hours for alcohol.

•Declaration of dry communities in the high prevalent regions.

•Promoting low strength alcohol for sale.

•Quality control of locally produced alcohol.

•Timely enforcement of legislation with penalties for violation of policy.

3. Strict border control for illegal importation

•Ban illegal importation through the porous border.

•Enforce punishment for the violators.

•Regulate entry of the duty-free alcohol into the country.

•Timely enforcement of legislation with penalties.

4. Age restriction

•Ban sale of alcohol to people under 18 years of age

5. Supporting prescriber and dispenser

•The strict control of prescription for restricted medications, such as opioid pain medication and benzodiazepines.

•Introduce electronic prescription to minimise dispensing errors and frauds.

•Coordinated online management of restricted medicines.

•Training and support of the prescriber and dispenser of restricted medicines.

•Developing National Guidelines for treatment of various addictive disorders.

6. Monitoring trend and data collection through ongoing research

8.4 Harm Reduction

Harm reduction refers to a whole range of public health policies aiming to reduce negative social and physical consequences of substance use disorder. It aims at the prevention of harm associated substance rather than prevention of drug itself. It aims at addressing the specific risk that arises from drug use. It promotes safe behaviour and minimises risk to the individuals, families, and communities. For example, drink driving laws, the needle exchange program, protecting children from the toxic drug-using environment. Availability of opioid substitution treatment (OST) in the community will minimise the risk of spreading blood-borne viruses.

1. Sobering up facility

•Non-custodial and safe overnight accommodation for publicly intoxicated people.

•It provides a bed, a meal, a shower, laundry facilities and other social support services.

•It can prevent public disruption and high-risk behaviour while severely intoxicated.

2. Safe transportation

•Mobile assistance patrols in the areas where people gather for drinking and using substances.

•Availability of public transport during events, and in the areas where people gather for drinking and using substance.

•Frequently checking Blood Alcohol levels of drivers.

3. Driving under intoxication

•Random alcohol and drug testing on drivers.

•Zero blood alcohol for drivers with provisional license.

•Severe penalties for the repeat offenders.

4. Safe event management

•Responsible venue operation

•Availability of free water in the venue

•Availability of emergency services

•Ensuring public safety in the venue

•Restricted supply of alcohol in the venue

5. Blood borne virus an STD prevention.

•Hep B vaccine

•STD testing, counselling, and treatment

•Counselling about safe use of needles

6. Safer injection practices

•Counselling about safe use of needles.

•Peer education about needle exchange program.

•Prevention and emergency response to overdose with naloxone.

•Medically supervised injection room and drug consumption room.

7. Substitution therapy

•Availability of medicines for opioid substitution therapy and other drugs (OST).

•Availability of OST centres in the remote areas.

8. High risk intervention

•Program for pregnant mothers to reduce use of substances during pregnancy.

•Programs for children of addicts.

9. Workforce

•Developing a multidisciplinary workforce to deliver preventative services, substitution therapies and responding to emergency situations.

All harm reduction strategies mentioned above are evidence-based, but some of them may not be relevant for development of drug policy for the remote region. However, the strategies mentioned below will be more specific to the remote and low resource setting regions of the developing countries. We can call them novel strategies.

Novel Harm Reduction Strategies for the low resource setting regions

•Employment generation for young addicts through Yunus Social Business model/social entrepreneurship.

•Making specific medication/substitution therapy available for substance withdrawals and craving in the remote community.

•Allocating some beds in the government general hospital in the remote community for treatment of addiction.

•Creating a register of the network of doctors in the local community for assessment and treatment of addiction and related health problems.

•Developing Telemedicine facility for consultation with the specialist from the city, and also to receive mentoring from the experienced addiction counsellors from the tertiary centres.

8.5 Pitfalls of current drug policy

Anecdotes, media, and political influence mainly drive the recent policy in India like many other nations. For drugs policy, it is easy to ignore the evidence-based approach and blame the individual for their choices. Hence, current policy is not developed around the requirement of grass root people and sadly it has ignored the significant effect of drugs on the family and children.

9.0 Clinical Aspect

9.1 Rehabilitation

Treatment of withdrawal symptoms is an important step towards recovery from addiction. Detoxification is not enough for sustained recovery. The recovery process of addiction is quite difficult and complex. The pathway of recovery involves elements of living skill, relapse prevention and substitution therapy. It involves helping people with the practical aspect of life, such as their living environment, employment opportunity, income source, and welfare of the family and their children. If all these issues are not addressed beforehand, substance use relapse is almost inevitable despite successful detoxification.

9.2 Brief intervention

Brief intervention is a short 5-15-minute targeted counselling session that reduces alcohol drinking in non-dependent drinkers in RCTs. The 'FLAGS' of brief intervention are as following:

Feedback- Provide individual feedback about the harm already caused by the substance in the individual and risks of future consequences due to ongoing use of the substance, including mental, physical, and social complications. For instance, substance abuse can cause poor sleep, lack of energy, poor concentration, weight loss, high blood pressure and injury to internal organs.

Listen- Actively listen to the patient and put their exact verbatim in the context while explaining current guideline about the safe level of use.

Advice- Provide concise and non-judgemental information about the importance of drinking pattern. Some examples of cutting down drinking include better sleep, more energy level, no hangover, better memory, improved concentration, improved mood, saving money, improving physical health parameters etc.

Goals- Encourage the patient to set a specific time-bound goal of their daily consumption of alcohol-based on safe drinking guideline.

Strategies:

Encourage the patient to develop some plans to achieve the goals. Some examples include drink only with solid food, drink a glass of water in between drinks, switching to smaller glass size, consume low alcohol content drink, avoid driving after drinking, keep a small amount of pocket money and allocate a specific time and place for drinking. Developing alternative pleasurable activities or coping strategies may minimise drinking if feeling bored and stressed out.

9.3 Identifying the substance use: CAGE

Excessive consumption of alcohol or any other substances for an extended period may cause dependence on the substance. Taking a drinking history usually requires a set of skills and strategies. The service provider needs to take a non-judgmental approach because blaming and criticising an individual usually makes people defensive and guarded.

Several evidence-based questionnaires can detect the problematic pattern of substance use. One easy to use questionnaire for the alcohol problem is an acronym of CAGE that requires two or more positive replies to identify problematic drinkers. C stands for cut down (Have you ever tried to cut down your alcohol drinking?).

A means annoyed (Have you ever been annoyed by your friend's and family's criticism of your drinking?). G stands for the guilty (Have you ever felt bad or guilty about your drinking). E stands for eye-opener (Have you ever felt shaky or hangover in the morning that you had to take a drink or two to get rid of that feeling?)

Similarly, specific questionnaires are available either to assess the severity of specific substance use or degree of withdrawal symptoms, such as AUDIT, ASSIST, AWS, SODQ, FNDQ etc. Scores generated from the scales provide clinicians with objective evidence of the severity of illness, which can be used as a reference point during recovery from illness.

9.4 The aim of substance use assessment

1. Understanding the use of substance in the context of an individual's life situation

2. Assessing severity of withdrawal symptoms

3. Understanding extent of psycho-social and physical health complication

4. Assessing risk taking behaviour

5. Determining 'Stage of motivation'

6. Previous abstinence attempts and the reason for relapse.

7. Assessing suitability for rehabilitation

8. Preventing relapse in future

9.5 Stages of change

Stage1 (precontemplation) – A substance dependent person in this stage does not see substance use as a problem. They decline all help with regards to treatment of substance use problem. Motivational interviewing techniques may be helpful at this stage.

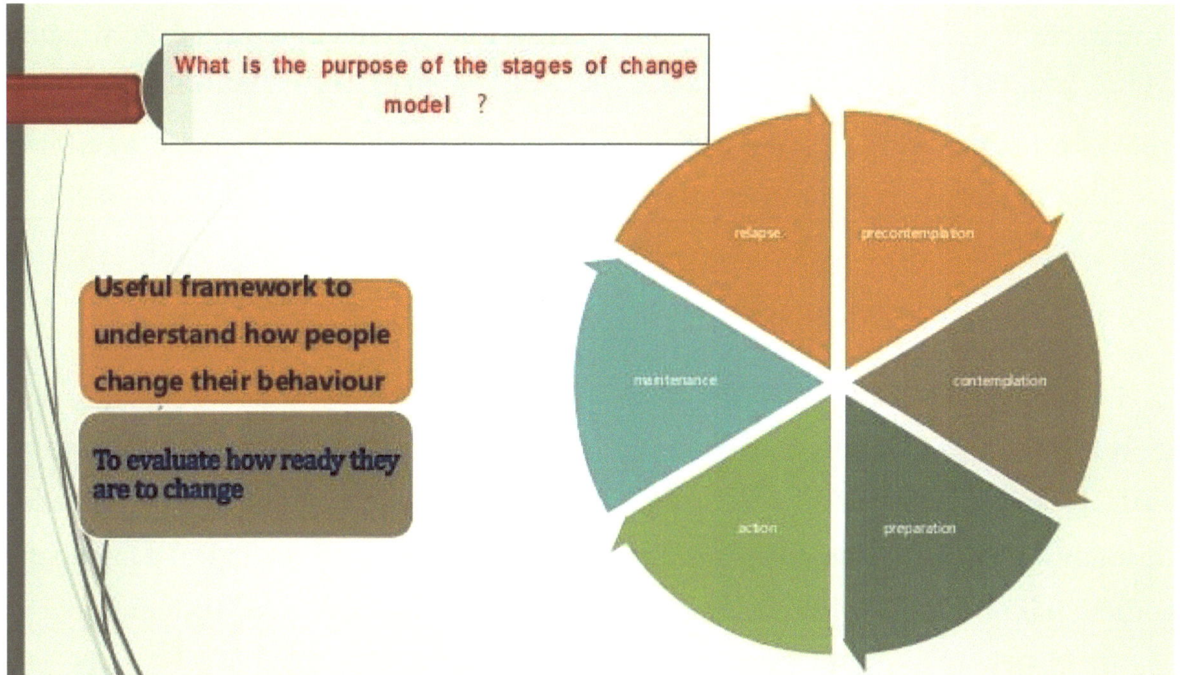

Figure 9.5.1

Stage2 (contemplation) – A substance dependent person in this stage is ambivalent or indecisive about the need for treatment. Motivational interviewing technique may be helpful.

Stage3 (preparation) – A substance dependent person in this stage is preparing to cut down or stop substance use. Goal setting strategies may be useful at this stage.

Stage 4(Action) – A substance dependent person in this stage has started taking active steps to cut down or stop substance use. Developing a treatment plan may be helpful at this stage.

Stage5 (maintenance) -**A** substance dependent person in this stage has successfully changed substance using habit and maintaining the abstinence. Relapse prevention strategies may be helpful.

9.6 Learning from the previous abstinence attempts

It is important to learn from the previous relapse what strategies worked to maintain abstinence and what might have gone wrong. An individual might notice that someone might have relapsed due to some triggering event after a sustained period of stability. These situations are called high-risk situations. Identifying high-risk situations by asking questions with 5Ws (when why where who what) usually helps identify skill deficits or coping skill deficits, leading to relapse.

9.7 Taking charge of addiction through goal setting

Total abstinence from a substance is not the only goal for the treatment of addiction. Focussing solely on abstinence will undermine the complexity of the addictive disorder. For example, an alcoholic person with significant physical and psychological damage due to addiction is not suitable for drinking in moderation. This group should rather strive for total abstinence. Goal setting is a crucial step. Every goal should be a SMART goal (specific, measurable, achievable, realistic, and time-bound). Short-term goals will lead to the long-term goal of total abstinence and reduce incidents of alcohol-related complications. For instance, reducing alcohol drinking to a safe level may decrease alcohol-related complications in the long-run.

9.8 Motivational interviewing

When most substance-dependent persons enter addiction treatment, they usually minimise their problems. Motivational interviewing helps them to navigate through their denial about the negative consequences of addiction. Motivational interviewing is undertaken in a non-judgemental manner by a trained person. It helps people weigh up good things and less good things about addiction and work through the ambivalence about seeking treatment for an addiction problem. The individual's personal decision-making process is reinforced by asking an open-ended and specific question about addiction's impact. The basic elements of motivational interviewing are:

- Expressing empathy through non-judgmental listening.
- Developing discrepancy between the client's goals and values with regards to their current behaviour.
- Rolling with resistance by avoiding arguments and confrontation.
- Eliciting client's own motivation for change.

Supporting client's self-efficacy brings change and sustain it as well.

9.9 Psychological therapy

It is an incredibly challenging to get a psychologist in a low resource setting in India. However, some self-help type of psychological strategies can be useful even in the geographically disadvantaged settings. Most evidence-based psychological therapies used in addiction treatment are cognitive behaviour therapy (CBT), contingency management (CM) and communication and assertiveness therapy. CBT entails identification of negative and unhelpful thought pattern and substituting it with more positive and problem-solving thoughts. CM entails positive reinforcement for desired behaviour, for instance, rewards for reduction of amount of substance use. Assertiveness skills may include drink refusal and learning to 'Say NO' through role-playing before implementing it in a real-life situation.

9.10 Medications for maintenance phase

After detoxification from a substance, maintenance medication therapy is required to prevent craving and propensity for relapse. For the opioid group of substances, there are two types of maintenance treatment: agonist maintenance and antagonist maintenance.

Methadone and buprenorphine are used for agonist maintenance, and naltrexone is used for antagonist maintenance. Most of the people would require agonist maintenance for a duration of months to years. Some people may need more prolonged maintenance treatment. During the maintenance phase, a recovering addict tries to modify their lifestyle, and they build up a healthy and supportive social network. After achieving some psychosocial stability, agonist medication can be gradually reduced and stopped. On the other hand, antagonist maintenance is usually indicated for highly motivated clients and people with a relatively shorter substance use duration.

Unfortunately, the availability of these medications is a major challenge in the remote Indian region. Methadone has serious side effects, such as breathing problem, disturbances of heart rhythm and accidental overdose. Opioids agonists can also be illegally traded off in the street if they are not administered under close supervision. All these factors make it difficult to prescribe specific medications for addictive disorder in the remote Indian community.

Naltrexone, despite being a relatively safe medication, is not preferred by the most addicts and dropout rate of naltrexone program is quite high. Additionally, naltrexone is a quite expensive medication and is not readily available in the remote Indian regions.

The dose of methadone is 30mg to 60 mg a day; it is generally started with a small dose and then built up to the maximum dose over a period of weeks to months. The rapid escalation of the dose may result in respiratory depression, cardiac arrhythmia and over sedation. Buprenorphine has an identical side effect profile compared to methadone, but buprenorphine is relatively safer in terms of respiratory depression and other side effects.

In terms of alcohol addiction, three types of medications are used for maintenance, such as disulfiram, acamprosate and naltrexone. Disulfiram is an aversive agent; people may have a serious reaction if they drink alcohol while taking it. Two other medications used for alcohol dependence are costly and not readily available in the remote region.

The dose of naltrexone is 50mg daily; the common side effects is hepatic dysfunction and nausea. Acamprosate is prescribed with 666mg thrice a day; a common side effect is a diarrhoea. Both medications are generally well tolerated. More recently, some new evidence is coming up about topiramate as well.

Medication	Dose	Maintenance	Side effects	Route of administration	Treatment
Methadone **mu receptor agonist**	Initial dose 5 mg -10 mg, gradually increased by 5-10mg every weekly, reaching 60mg in 4-6 weeks. Maximum dose is 100mg a day	Opioids drugs	*Sedation, QTC prolongation (higher dosage >80mg a day), respiratory depression, nausea, and constipation*	Tablet and oral solution. Supervised dispensing.	Variable Generally, lasts for years
Buprenorphine **(Subutex)** **Kappa receptor, partial agonist**	Initial dose 1-2mg a day, gradually increasing to 12 mg a day. Some patients may need higher dosage	Opioid drugs	*Sedation, QTc prolongation, constipation, dizziness nausea, decreased libido hypotension.*	Buprenorphine (Subutex) Kappa receptor, partial agonist	Initial dose 1-2mg a day, gradually increasing to 12 mg a day. Some patients may need higher dosage

	up to 16mg.		*Respiratory depression may happen but less common.*		up to 16mg.
Buprenorphine-naloxone combination(subox one) **Prevents overdose if injected**	As above	Opioid drugs	*As above*	sublingual	Months to years
Naltrexone **Antagonist for all opioid receptors**	50 mg a day Or twice weekly dispense	Opioids drugs and anti-craving for alcohol dependence	*Headache, pain, nausea, insomnia, and mood changes*	tablet	Months to years
Acamprosate **NMDA receptor**	333mg tablet Two tablets TDS if body weight is >60kg and 4 tablets in divided dosage if body weight	Alcohol dependence, reduces craving and reverses brain chemistry caused by chronic alcohol use.	*Nausea, vomiting, diarrhoea, headache, and insomnia*	tablet	Months to years

	is <60kg.				
Disulfiram **Aversive agent**	250-500mg a day	Alcohol dependence syndrome	*Antabuse reaction when alcohol is consumed with disulfiram* *(throbbing headache, vomiting, hypertension, flushing, fainting, and dizziness)*	tablet	Months to years

Table 9.10.1

9.11 Craving management

Craving is inevitable during the early days of abstinence. Craving can be triggered by some specific emotional events, which could be either a positive event, such as celebration or negative events such as low mood and stress. It is important to educate clients that craving is a temporary phenomenon, and it will subside soon, just like a wave in the ocean. Evidence suggests that people can deal with craving by using 3Ds approach (distraction, decision, and delay). This is called urge surfing. Some medication can help with craving, for instance, Naltrexone for alcohol craving.

9.12 Relapse prevention

Substance use disorder is a chronic relapsing condition. It is unrealistic to think that detoxification will lead to abstinence form substance. While successful management of substance withdrawal symptoms may contain the physiological aspect of addiction, it cannot replenish the skill deficits required to prevent relapse. Relapse prevention strategies empower an addict to develop skills to deal with craving for substance use in high-risk situations. A little slip-up can be quite devastating for a recovering addict, which often leads to full-blown relapse. Relapse is generally a learning experience for an individual, and every slip-up allows them to identify potential causes for relapse. It reminds them to reintroduce all previously useful strategies which helped them to maintain sobriety. Maintaining a substance use diary may help identify triggers for relapse, and it also may activate some relapse prevention strategies to prevent a full-blown relapse.

9.13 Social reinforcement

Substance use can be a symptom of underlying social and economic disadvantage. All these issues need to be addressed to achieve sustained recovery from addiction. Long term substance use can drive a person into social disadvantage, marginalisation, and poverty. Hence, substance rehabilitation program usually aims at building up community living skill, developing a sense of self-responsibility, and sharpening of interpersonal skill. Social reinforcement activities may also help to establish supportive social network. It can encourage the individuals to develop healthy lifestyle and finding out pleasures in alternative activities. Social reinforcement may also facilitate some employment opportunities in various locally sustainable activities.

9.14 Peer Support Network

Good peer support network of recovering addicts can boast their confidence, and it can instill hope in the new entrants. The support network can also help people when they are at the verge of relapse. Additionally, family members of addicts can develop a network among themselves and exchange their own personal experiences through mutual sharing and support. Peer support group can minimise the sense of isolation, stigma, and cultivate a sense of belonging. One example of peer support group is alcohol anonymous. Research has shown that influence of peer support group can be disseminated to the larger community for better outcome.

9.15 Therapeutic community

Therapeutic community is a more democratic environment than typical residential drug rehabilitation centres. A therapeutic community is being run by recovering addicts. It is bound by strict ground rules. Residents of a therapeutic community learn daily living skills through mutual sharing and role modelling. Every client is identified only by their names. All residents in the therapeutic community are required to do certain basic tasks daily. New entrants to the community learn from the senior members through observation and role modelling. Mutual respect and coordination between members remain the crucial aspect for the smooth functioning of the therapeutic community. Additionally, community members have an opportunity to learn certain vocational skill through supervised activities. While remaining in the community, the recovering addicts re-establish their connection with the family and friends who do not have issues with addiction. After a period of 3-6 months, a community member gradually proceeds towards graduation from the therapeutic community. After leaving therapeutic community, the ex-members still can contribute to the recovery of current members by participating in different activities in the therapeutic community. After graduating from the therapeutic community, an ex-member can also develop a peer support network in the community to identify new clients and support their families.

10.0 Management of substance use disorder in low resource setting

Substance use disorder patients presenting in the low resource setting of India are unique. Their nature of presentation and source of referral is quite different. Additionally, addiction treatment facilities are scarce in the remote low resource setting of India. A handful of psychiatrists, whoever is practising in the remote region, usually find the treatment of substance dependence difficult due to non-availability of specific medications, lack of the trained workforce, and scarce treatment facilities. Treatment of substance use disorder usually involves teamwork and integrated approach. Allied health professionals play a pivotal role in the recovery of substance dependence. Patients rarely visit a doctor directly for the treatment of addiction. Their family member usually brings them for treatment. They may be incidentally diagnosed when they are visiting a local doctor for other health problems. As substance use problem often starts at a young age, local high schools and colleges can be a good source of addiction clients; but patients are rarely referred from those educational institutions. Addiction patients are seldom referred from the legal services for the mandatory treatment of substance use disorder. Thus, source of referral is quite restricted in the remote regions of India.

People of the remote region has a limited awareness about the illness model of addiction. They often consider addiction as a personal weakness or moral problem. A substance-dependent individual is usually ostracised by the small community of the remote region in India because vast majority of people living there are teetotallers. In addition to addicts, their family members also suffer a lot because they are often being criticised and discriminated by society. Remote regions of India, which are deprived of even basic health care facilities, treatment of addictive disorder remains their lowest priority issue. Interestingly, you do not require a super modern medical centre for treatment of addiction, because an addictive disorder can be managed even in the primary health care facilities by local doctors if they have some supervision and training.

Whatever the source of referral, as soon as a patient with addiction comes through the door for treatment of addiction in the remote low resource regions of India, the local doctors must have some strategies in their mind, they must know the way of approaching this group in their clinic.

We have formulated a seven-step strategy to highlight what a doctor working in the remote and low resource setting Indian region should do when a patient with addiction comes through their door.s

First Step- A doctor will need to know all concerns and expectations of the patient and the referrer. It is essential to organise a though physical examination, the baseline blood tests and ECG. An internal medicine doctor must be involved if there are any major concerns about physical health.

Second Step-The local doctor needs to gather the history of addiction in terms of amount, frequency, and severity of use. They can wisely utilise the consultation time to conduct a session of brief intervention, which is a short 5-15-minute targeted counselling session shown to reduce alcohol drinking in non-dependent drinkers in RCTs. Brief intervention does not need any specialised training, and it is so simple that any health professional can do it.

Third Step- This step will entail an assessment of motivation, and the reason for motivation by using Readiness to Change Questionnaire. The score of the questionnaire is divided into pre-contemplation, contemplation, and action. The total score will determine their level of motivation.

Fourth Step- There are three components, such as conducting a thorough mental state examination, assessment of risk to self or others and deciding on the treatment setting. Patients who are expressing suicidal thoughts should be treated in the psychiatric inpatient facility. A psychiatrist must be involved because patients might have some underlying mental illness. As there is a dearth of psychiatric treatment facilities in the remote region, it is prudent to explain family members about risk, and it is better to refer them to a tertiary centre if the risk is imminent.

Fifth Step- This step involves detoxification from the substance. Detoxification starts with an assessment of the severity of withdrawal symptoms, both clinically and using some rating scales. The withdrawal symptoms score derived from the scale can help the clinician to optimise the dosage of medication. This stage is called detoxification. People can detoxify themselves from a substance in the Detox centre or through home-based treatment. Some less severely affected people end up in doing Cold Turkey method. Inpatient detox is always better than the outpatient/community detox. In the remote Indian towns, inpatient detox can only be done in the general hospital ward if hospital authority allows doing that. Substance detoxification is a risky affair, and it should not be taken lightly. A pathway must be established beforehand so that complicated detox patient can be immediately referred.

Red flag signs during detox

Seizure

Difficulties in breathing

Confusing due to over-sedation

Severely decreased or increased heart rate.

Signs of delirium tremens

Severe GI upset during withdrawal.

Suicidal patient

Severe electrolyte abnormalities and nutritional deficiency

Any of these red flag signs will alert the clinician to transfer the patient to a general hospital as per established pathway set out beforehand.

Sixth Step- Treatment of addiction is not only involved removing the substance from the body, but it also involves extensive psychological and social rehabilitation. Degree of the social impact of addiction can be assessed by using a scale named Addiction Severity Index (ASI). After that, psychosocial goals can be gradually achieved by using rewards and reinforcement. Substance rehabilitation is a highly structured and sophisticated process of recovery. Rehabilitation usually starts in the confined space of the rehabilitation centre. The strict ground rules bound the environment in the substance rehabilitation centre. That is why many patients do not prefer rehabilitation of addiction. Additionally, the substance rehab program is typically run by a team of allied health professionals, such as social worker, nurse, counsellor, and psychologist. It is nearly impossible to get such a specialised group of professionals in the remote and low resource setting. Local health professionals can undertake some short-term training in this matter, and they can work as a facilitator of the group in the rehab program. Furthermore, all ex-clients can offer some contribution as a facilitator to the rehab group. The local doctor needs to be aware of different substance rehabilitation centres in the region, and they should refer patients to appropriate centres if necessary.

Step Seven- Substance dependence is a chronic relapsing condition. People usually take multiple attempts before achieving total abstinence from the substance. Momentary lapse to substance use should not be demonised. Every relapse should be considered as a learning experience. Recovering addicts should undertake some relapse prevention counselling to alleviate the risk of relapse. This is probably the hardest thing to achieve in the remote Indian region. Previously recovered peers or local deaddiction centres will be able to provide this type of counselling.

11.0 TERMINOLOGY IN ADDICTIVE DISORDER

There are many medical jargons frequently used in addictive disorder, which needs be clarified for the public and non-specialists.

i. **Tolerance**- means increasing amount of substance consumption to have the same effect/buzz. It is a common pattern in substance use disorder that it starts with a small amount of consumption, eventually requiring a large amount of substance to have the same effect. Our body becomes habituated to the substance due to neuroadaptation.

ii. **Craving**- means an overpowering desire to use substance, which is preceded by immense psychological and physical discomfort.

iii. **Salience-** A great deal of time is spent from procuring substance, remaining under influence of substance, and recovering from substance.

iv. **Lapse-** 'Little slip up' or recommencement of substance use after a period of abstinence.

v. **Relapse-** Retuning to   full blown or previous level of substance abuse after a period of abstinence. It is usually preceded by a lapse.

vi. **Reinstatement-** Tendency to rapid reversal to the previous level of substance use when someone relapses after a period of abstinence due to upregulation of brain receptors.

vii. **Paraphernalia-** all equipment required for substance use activities. For example, syringes used for intravenous illicit drug. Drug using people make different makeshift equipment to facilitate their drug using habit.

12.0 Appendix

Rating scale to assess the severity of substance use disorder

1. Severity of alcohol dependence questionnaire- measures severity of alcohol drinking over last 6 months. Source-https://smartcjs.org.uk/professionals/gps/screening-tools/

2. Alcohol withdrawal scale (CIWA-Ar) - measures alcohol withdrawal symptoms. Source-https://smartcjs.org.uk/professionals/gps/screening-tools/

3. Alcohol use disorder identification test (AUDIT)-measures whether there are any problems with alcohol drinking. Source-https://smartcjs.org.uk/professionals/gps/screening-tools/

4. Severity of opiate dependence questionnaire (SODQ)- measures severity of opiate dependence. Source-https://smartcjs.org.uk/professionals/gps/screening-tools/

5. Severity of dependence scale (SDS)- measures severity of substance dependence

6. Diary of alcohol drinking- source- https://pubs.niaa.nih.gov/handout

7. Fagerstorm Nicotine dependence Scale (FNDS)- measures nicotine dependence. Source- https://smartcjs.org.uk/professionals/gps/screening-tools/

8. Amphetamine withdrawal questionnaire.

 Source-https://smartcjs.org.uk/professionals/gps/screening-tools/

9. CIWA-B- for benzodiazepine withdrawal symptoms-.

 Source-https://smartcjs.org.uk/professionals/gps/screening-tools/

10. Alcohol Smoking Substance Involvement Screening Tool (ASSIST) - screening for all substances followed by recommendation what to do. World Health organisation.

11. Drug Abuse Screening Test (DAST) - for screening of all types of substances apart from nicotine and alcohol. Source-https://www.who.int/assist

12. Addiction Severity Index (ASI)- for severity of addiction and its psychosocial complications.www.bu.edu › igsw › online-courses › substanceabuse.

13. Readiness to Change Questionnaire. - for assessment of someone's motivation.

13.0 Reference

1. Cacace, M., Ettelt, S., Mays, N., & Nolte, E. (2013). Assessing quality in cross-country comparisons of health systems and policies: Towards a set of generic quality criteria. *Health policy, 112*(1-2), 156-162. doi:10.1016/j.healthpol.2013.03.020

2. Demirkol,A(2011).Problem drinking management in general parctice. Australian family Physician,40(8),576-582.

3. Dhawan,A, Rao, R, Ambekar, A, Pusp, A & Ray, R(2017). Treatment of substance use disorder through the governemnt health facilities: Developments in the "Drug De-addiction Programme" of Ministry of Health and Family Welfare,Government of India. Indian Journal of Psychiatry,59(3),380-384.

4. drugfacts@nida.nih.gov

5. Ford, B. A. (2013). From mountains to molehills: a comparative analysis of drug policy. *Annual Survey of International & Comparative Law, 19*(1), 197-231.

6. Gillespie, N. (2009). Drug Decriminalization in Portugal. *Reason, 41*(3), 13.

7. Gowing, L., Proudfoot, H., Henry-Edwards, S., & Teesson, M. (2001). *Evidence supporting treatment.*

Hamilton, G., Cross, D., Resnicow, K., & Shaw, T. (2007). Does harm minimisation lead to greater experimentation? Results from a school smoking intervention trial. *Drug and Alcohol Review, 26*(6), 605-613.

8. Hudoba, M., Grenyer, B. F. S., & O'Toole, M. (2004). Development of an enhanced needle and syringe programme: the First Step programme pilot. *Drug and Alcohol Review, 23*(3), 295-297. doi:10.1080/09595230412331289455

9. Hughes C, & Stevens A. . (2007). The Effects of Decriminalization of Drug Use in Portugal,   .
https://www.academia.edu/270213/The_Effects_of_the_Decriminalization_of_Drug_Use_In_Portugal

10. Hughes, C. E., & Stevens, A. (2012). A resounding success or a disastrous failure: Re-examining the interpretation of evidence on the Portuguese decriminalisation of illicit drugs. *Drug and Alcohol Review, 31*(1), 101-113. doi:10.1111/j.1465-

3362.2011.00383.x Jackson NJ, Isen JD, Khoddam R, et al. Impact of adolescent marijuana use on intelligence: Results from two longitudinal twin studies. Proc Natl Acad Sci U S A. 2016;113(5):E500-E508. doi:10.1073/pnas.1516648113.

11. Jarvis,TTebbut,J. & Mattick,R.P.(1995).Treatment approaches for alcohol and drug dependence: An introductory guide.Sydney: Wiley & Sons.

12. Proudfoot H; Henry-Edwards S & Teesson M. Evidence supporting treatment: the effectiveness of interventions for illicit drug use. ANCD Research Paper 3. Canberra: Australian National CouncilonDrugs,2001.https://www.researchgate.net/publication/281834004_E vidence_supporting_treatment.

13. Marlatt,G.A. & Gordon,J.(1985).Relapse prevention:Maintenance stragies in the treatment of addictive behaviour.NY:Guldford Press.

14. Marmor, T. R. (2017). Comparative Studies and the Drawing of Policy Lessons: Describing, Explaining, Evaluating, and Predicting. *Journal of Comparative Policy Analysis: Research and Practice, 19*(4), 313-326. doi:10.1080/13876988.2017.1279439

15. Mattick,R.P. & Hall,W.(1994).A summary of the recommendations for the management of opioid dependence:The quality assurance in the treatment of drug dependence project.Drug and Alcohol Review,13,319-326.

16. Mattick R.P. & Hall,W.(1994). A summary of recommendations for the management of alcohol problems: The quality assurance in the treatment of drug dependence project.Drug and Alcohol Review13,145-155.

17. Miller,W.R. & Rollnick,S(2002).Motivational Interviewing:Preparaing people to change addictive behaviour(2nd Ed.).New ork:Guldford Press.

18. Poduthase, H., & J Vellappally, A. (2016). *Alcohol Policies in India and United States: A Comparative Policy Analysis* (Vol. 1).

19. Ritter, A. (2010). Illicit drugs policy through the lens of regulation. *International Journal of Drug Policy, 21*(4), 265-270. doi:https://doi.org/10.1016/j.drugpo.2009.11.002

20. Ritter, A., & Cameron, J. (2006). A review of the efficacy and effectiveness of harm reduction strategies for alcohol, tobacco and illicit drugs. *Drug and Alcohol Review, 25*(6), 611-624.

21. Rosenfeld, R., & Decker, S. H. (1999). Are arrest statistics a valid measure of illicit drug use? The relationship between criminal justice and public health indicators of cocaine, heroin, and marijuana use. *Justice Quarterly : JQ, 16*(3), 685-699. doi:10.1080/07418829900094311

22. Tracy,K &Wallace,P,S(2016). benefits of peer support group in treatment of addiction.Substabce abuse and rehabilitation,7:143-154

23. The national drug dependence and treatment centre. (2018). Magnitute of Substance Use in India Retrieved 3/04/19, from Ministy of social justice and empowerment government of India http://164.100.117.97/WriteReadData/userfiles/Exec-Sum_For%20Media.pdf

24. Wellbourne-Wood, D. (1999). Harm reduction in Australia: some problems putting policy into practice. *International Journal of Drug Policy, 10*(5), 403-413. doi:10.1016/S0955-3959(99)00037-7

25. White, B., Haber, P. S., & Day, C. A. (2016). Community attitudes towards harm reduction services and a newly established needle and syringe automatic dispensing machine in an inner-city area of Sydney, Australia. *The International Journal on Drug Policy, 27*, 121. doi:10.1016/j.drugpo.2015.05.010

26. World Health Organization. Disorders due to substance use. *WHO Mental Health Gap Action Programme (mhGAP).* Retrieved from https://www.who.int/mental_health/mhgap/sub_supporting_material.pdf?ua=1